The Athlete's Trip

Unleashing the Potential of Magic Mushrooms for Athletic Performance

By True Eira
Ancient Wisdom for Modern Healing

Visit
trueeira.com/test
Find Your Microdose Personality

TRUE
EIRA

ABOUT AUTHOR

Travis Eric, spearheading the research initiatives at True Eira, is a seasoned expert in the cultivation of mushrooms and a leader in microdosing for athletic performance. With a deep understanding of the nuances of various strains, Travis offers a unique, grassroots level of expertise. This knowledge is complemented by the diverse experiences of the True Eira team, combining scientific rigor with practical application. Together, they have explored microdoseing across various athletic disciplines, engaging with athletes ranging from hockey players and long-distance runners to competition-level bodybuilders. This extensive exploration has provided invaluable insights into the practical effects of these substances on physical and mental performance.

In "The Athlete's Trip," the collective wisdom of Travis and the True Eira team is distilled into a comprehensive guide. Their work transcends traditional approaches, offering a holistic view that melds the physical, mental, and spiritual aspects of athletic performance. The book is a testament to their dedication to enhancing athletic performance through innovative, informed, and responsible use of microdosing and other holistic practices. Their collaborative efforts aim to illuminate the path for athletes and fitness enthusiasts who seek to push the boundaries of their capabilities and achieve peak performance.

TRUE
EIRA

Visit

trueeira.com/test

Find Your Microdose Personality

**TRUE
EIRA**

Table of Contents

True Eira

Ancient Wisdom for Modern Healing

Visit

trueeira.com/test

Find Your Microdose Personality

TRUE
EIRA

Introduction

In today's fiercely competitive sports and fitness world, athletes constantly seek innovative ways to gain an edge and unlock their full athletic potential. As the boundaries of human performance continue to be pushed, an unexpected ally has emerged from the realm of ancient wisdom and cutting-edge research: magic mushrooms.

Harnessing the power of these natural psychedelic substances, athletes and fitness enthusiasts are exploring a revolutionary approach to optimizing their physical and mental performance. But how can something traditionally associated with spiritual and introspective journeys be the key to unlocking new levels of strength, endurance, and mental resilience?

Welcome to the world of microdosing and macrodosing magic mushrooms for athletic performance. This book will take you on a thrilling exploration of the untapped potential of psychedelics as performance enhancers, delving into the science, personal stories, and practical applications of this groundbreaking approach.

With growing research and anecdotal evidence supporting the role of psychedelics in improving focus, creativity, and mental well-being, it's no wonder that athletes are turning to these powerful substances to overcome barriers and reach new heights. Whether you're a professional athlete, a dedicated gym-goer, or simply someone interested in exploring the frontiers of human potential, this book will open your eyes to the astonishing possibilities within the realm of psychedelic-enhanced performance.

Embark on this exhilarating journey with us as we uncover the secrets of magic mushrooms and their ability to transform how we approach athletic performance. We'll delve into microdosing and macrodosing and the synergistic effects of combining these powerful substances with other performance-enhancing practices. Along the way, we'll demystify the science, share personal experiences, and provide practical guidance for those looking to incorporate these potent allies into their performance-enhancing routines.

Join us as we unveil the extraordinary potential of magic mushrooms in the pursuit of peak athletic performance, and discover how you, too, can tap into this ancient wisdom to unlock your full potential.

The Potential of Magic Mushrooms for Athletic Performance

The world of athletics has long been fascinated by the quest for peak performance, constantly seeking innovative methods to push the limits of human potential. In recent years, an unexpected contender has emerged as a powerful ally in this pursuit: magic mushrooms. These naturally occurring psychedelic substances, containing the active compound psilocybin, have shown remarkable promise in enhancing various aspects of athletic performance.

While magic mushrooms have been traditionally associated with spiritual and reflective experiences, a growing body of research and anecdotal evidence suggests that they can also positively impact physical and mental performance in athletes. Magic mushrooms can enable athletes to tap into previously unexplored realms of their abilities by fostering heightened focus, mental clarity, and resilience.

From endurance sports to strength training and everything in between, magic mushrooms can revolutionize how athletes approach their training and competition. By harnessing the unique properties of psilocybin, athletes can unlock new levels of motivation, overcome mental barriers, and cultivate a deep connection with their bodies and minds.

In this book, we will explore the potential of magic mushrooms as a powerful tool for athletic performance enhancement. We will delve into the science behind their effects, discuss how they can optimize physical and mental performance, and provide an overview of the exciting possibilities as more athletes and researchers explore this untapped potential.

Microdosing and Macrodosing Explained

To understand the potential of magic mushrooms for athletic performance enhancement, it is essential first to comprehend the concepts of microdosing and macrodosing. These two methods of using magic mushrooms differ significantly in dosage and intended effects, making them suitable for different purposes within an athlete's training regimen.

Microdosing: Microdosing involves the consumption of a sub-perceptual dose of magic mushrooms, typically between 0.1 to 0.3 grams. At such low doses, the psychedelic effects of the mushrooms are not experienced, but their subtle cognitive and emotional benefits can still be felt. Athletes who choose to microdose may report improved focus, mental clarity, increased creativity, and reduced anxiety, all of which can contribute to enhanced athletic performance. Microdosing is typically practiced on a schedule, like once every three days, to maintain the desired effects without building tolerance.

Macrodosing: Macrodosing, on the other hand, refers to the consumption of a full psychedelic dose of magic mushrooms, usually ranging between 2 to 5 grams or more. This dosage results in a potent psychedelic experience that can last for several hours, inducing profound shifts in perception, emotion, and cognition. While macrodosing is not typically used as a direct performance-enhancing strategy during training or competition, it can still provide valuable insights for athletes. The reflective nature of a macrodosing experience may help athletes confront mental blocks, develop a stronger mind-body connection, or gain a deeper understanding of their motivations and goals.

Both microdosing and macrodosing have unique applications within the context of athletic performance enhancement. By understanding the differences between these two methods and how they can be strategically implemented, athletes can harness the full potential of magic mushrooms to optimize their physical and mental performance.

The Role of Psychedelics in Optimizing Physical and Mental Performance

Psychedelics, such as magic mushrooms, have been gaining increasing attention in recent years for their potential to enhance physical and mental performance. While the use of psychedelics in sports and fitness may seem unconventional, growing evidence suggests that these substances can provide valuable benefits to athletes when used responsibly and strategically.

Mental performance: One of the primary ways psychedelics can contribute to enhanced performance is through their effects on mental well-being and cognitive function. Many athletes experience mental barriers, such as performance anxiety, self-doubt, or a lack of motivation, which can hinder their progress and success. Psychedelics have been shown to promote self-reflection, increased self-awareness, and improved emotional regulation, helping athletes overcome these psychological obstacles. Moreover, microdosing has been associated with increased creativity, focus, and cognitive flexibility, which can lead to innovative training strategies and better decision-making in competitions.

Mind-body connection: Psychedelics, particularly during macrodosing experiences, can facilitate a stronger mind-body connection, enabling athletes to develop a deeper understanding of their physical capabilities and limitations. This enhanced connection can lead to improved body awareness, more efficient movement patterns, and a greater ability to listen to and interpret the body's signals, resulting in reduced injury risk and optimized performance

Recovery and resilience: Research has shown that psychedelics, such as magic mushrooms, can help reduce symptoms of anxiety, depression, and post-traumatic stress disorder (PTSD). For athletes facing mental health challenges or struggling with the psychological impact of injuries, psychedelics may provide a valuable tool for promoting mental resilience and accelerating recovery.

Flow states: Psychedelics have been linked to the experience of "flow" – a mental state characterized by complete immersion in an activity, where time seems to slow down and a sense of effortless control is felt. Achieving a flow state can lead to peak performance in sports, enabling athletes to operate at the highest levels of skill, concentration, and confidence.

The responsible and strategic use of psychedelics, such as magic mushrooms, can significantly optimize athletes' physical and mental performance. By harnessing the unique benefits of these substances, athletes may unlock new levels of potential and achieve tremendous success in their chosen sports.

Overview of the Book's Content

This comprehensive book explores the potential benefits and applications of magic mushrooms in the realm of athletic performance, with a focus on both physical and mental aspects. Beginning with examining the science behind magic mushrooms and their effects on the brain and body, we delve into a wide range of topics, including the role of serotonin in athletic performance and the impact of neuroplasticity on training and recovery.

We provide practical advice on microdosing and macrodosing, explaining their benefits and applications for athletes, such as enhanced focus, improved mood, increased physical endurance, and faster recovery. The book also investigates the potential for combining magic mushrooms with other performance enhancers, covering both legal and illegal substances, and the synergistic effects that may arise from such combinations.

Moreover, we explore the world of mindfulness practices, such as meditation, breathwork, and yoga, discussing their potential to enhance athletic performance and complement the use of magic mushrooms. Emphasizing the importance of a personalized and holistic approach, we discuss how to integrate magic mushrooms into an existing training regimen, balance physical, mental, and emotional well-being, and develop an adaptable plan to track progress and make adjustments as needed.

We also address the role of sleep and recovery in athletic performance, exploring the potential influence of magic mushrooms on sleep quality and recovery and the connection between sleep, training, and psychedelic use. Furthermore, the book examines the mental aspects of athletic performance, including techniques to develop mental toughness, resilience, and a growth mindset.

The book touches upon injury prevention, pain management, and the potential benefits of microdosing and macrodosing for injury recovery. Additionally, we discuss the ethical and legal considerations surrounding using magic mushrooms for performance enhancement, covering topics such as sportsmanship, fair competition, and the role of governing bodies and anti-doping agencies.

Throughout the book, we share real-life examples and case studies to inspire athletes and fitness enthusiasts to explore the potential of magic mushrooms responsibly and informally. Finally, we look at the future of psychedelics in sports and training and provide resources for further exploration, including books, articles, websites, workshops, and professional organizations.

The Science Behind Magic Mushrooms

This chapter will uncover the fascinating science behind magic mushrooms and how they can potentially revolutionize athletic performance. We will begin by examining the primary psychedelic compounds present in magic mushrooms, psilocybin, and psilocin, which are responsible for the mind-altering effects of these fungi. Understanding their chemical makeup will give you insight into how these substances interact with the brain and body.

Next, we will delve into the role of serotonin, a key neurotransmitter in regulating mood, appetite, sleep, and more. You'll learn about the connection between serotonin and athletic performance and how magic mushrooms can influence serotonin levels in the brain. This knowledge will help you appreciate the broader implications of using magic mushrooms in the context of sports and physical training.

Moreover, we will explore the concept of neuroplasticity, which refers to the brain's ability to reorganize itself by forming new neural connections throughout life. Neuroplasticity plays a crucial role in learning, adaptation, and recovery, making it an essential aspect of athletic training. We will discuss how magic mushrooms can enhance neuroplasticity, providing a solid foundation for you to incorporate these powerful substances into your athletic pursuits.

By the end of this chapter, you will have a comprehensive understanding of the scientific principles underlying magic mushrooms and their potential applications in sports and physical performance. Armed with this knowledge, you'll be better equipped to make informed decisions about integrating these substances into your training regimen and maximizing their benefits for your athletic goals.

Psychedelic Compounds: Psilocybin and Psilocin

Magic mushrooms, also known as psilocybin mushrooms, contain two primary psychedelic compounds: psilocybin and psilocin. These compounds are responsible for the mind-altering effects commonly associated with magic mushrooms.

Psilocybin is a prodrug, which is metabolized in the body and converted into its active form, psilocin. When consumed, psilocybin is quickly dephosphorylated by liver enzymes, resulting in psilocin formation. Once psilocin is present in the bloodstream, it can cross the blood-brain barrier and interact with the brain's neurotransmitter system, specifically binding to serotonin receptors.

The psychoactive effects of psilocin stem from its ability to bind to serotonin 2A (5-HT2A) receptors in the brain. This interaction leads to a cascade of neural activity, resulting in the psychedelic experience characterized by alterations in perception, cognition, and emotions. These effects can vary greatly depending on the dosage, individual factors, and the context in which the magic mushrooms are consumed.

Understanding the chemical makeup of psilocybin and psilocin and their interactions with the brain is essential for appreciating the potential of magic mushrooms in the context of athletic performance and personal growth. In the following sections, we will explore how these psychedelic compounds can influence various physical and mental performance aspects, providing a foundation for their potential applications in sports and training.

How Magic Mushrooms Affect the Brain and Body

Magic mushrooms have a profound impact on both the brain and the body, leading to various effects on athletic performance and overall well-being. The active compounds in magic mushrooms, psilocybin, and psilocin, primarily interact with the brain's serotonin system, influencing various cognitive and physiological functions.

When psilocin binds to serotonin 2A (5-HT2A) receptors in the brain, it triggers a series of events that result in the classic psychedelic experience. Some of the most notable effects of magic mushrooms on the brain include:

Altered perception: Users often report changes in visual, auditory, and tactile perception. Colors may appear more vibrant, sounds more pronounced, and the sense of touch may be heightened.

Enhanced creativity and cognitive flexibility: Magic mushrooms have been shown to increase connectivity between different brain regions, which can lead to improved problem-solving abilities, more fluid thinking, and heightened creativity.

Emotional and introspective experiences: Magic mushrooms can evoke emotions, from euphoria to anxiety, and can facilitate introspection and self-reflection. This can lead to personal growth and a deeper understanding of mental barriers or limitations.

In addition to these cognitive effects, magic mushrooms can also impact the body in several ways.

Increased heart rate and blood pressure: The stimulation of serotonin receptors can lead to increased cardiovascular activity. While this is typically safe for healthy individuals, it's essential to be aware of these physiological changes, especially for athletes.

Improved mind-body connection: Magic mushrooms can enhance body awareness and proprioception, which may translate to improved coordination, balance, and overall athletic performance.

Potential impact on the immune system: While more research is needed, some studies have suggested that psychedelics like magic mushrooms could have immunomodulatory effects, which may influence an athlete's recovery and overall health.

It's essential to recognize that the effects of magic mushrooms can vary greatly depending on the individual, dosage, and context in which they are consumed. As we explore the potential applications of magic mushrooms in athletic performance, it's crucial to consider these factors and approach their use responsibly and with an understanding of the possible risks and benefits.

The Role of Serotonin in Athletic Performance

Serotonin is a neurotransmitter that modulates various physiological and cognitive functions, including mood, appetite, sleep, and cognition. In the context of athletic performance, serotonin can significantly impact several aspects that contribute to an athlete's success.

Mood and motivation: Serotonin is often called the "feel-good" neurotransmitter, as it is closely associated with feelings of happiness and well-being. Adequate serotonin levels can lead to improved mood, increased motivation, and a more positive outlook, crucial for maintaining a consistent and effective training regimen.

Energy and fatigue: Serotonin regulates energy balance and can influence an athlete's perception of fatigue. High serotonin levels in the brain may contribute to central fatigue, a phenomenon where the brain signals the body to slow down or stop physical activity. On the other hand, low serotonin levels can result in a lack of motivation and energy, which can negatively impact training performance.

Sleep and recovery: Serotonin plays a key role in the regulation of sleep, as it is a precursor to melatonin, the hormone responsible for regulating sleep-wake cycles. Adequate sleep is crucial for athletes, allowing for proper recovery, muscle repair, and overall performance optimization. Serotonin's role in sleep regulation directly impacts an athlete's ability to recover from training and maintain peak performance.

Pain perception: Serotonin also plays a role in modulating pain perception. Higher serotonin levels can contribute to reduced pain sensitivity, which may help athletes push through discomfort during training and competitions. However, it's essential to maintain a balance and listen to the body's signals to avoid overtraining or injury.

Given the role of serotonin in these various aspects of athletic performance, it's no surprise that magic mushrooms, which primarily interact with the serotonin system, have garnered interest as potential performance-enhancing agents. However, it's essential to approach their use with caution, understanding, and a comprehensive knowledge of both the potential benefits and risks involved.

Neuroplasticity and its Impact on Training and Recovery

Neuroplasticity refers to the brain's ability to change and adapt to new experiences, learning, and environmental stimuli. This inherent flexibility allows the brain to reorganize neural connections, create new ones, and generate new neurons. Neuroplasticity is crucial in various athletic performance aspects, particularly training and recovery.

Skill acquisition and mastery: As athletes learn and practice new skills, the brain forms and strengthens neural connections to encode and retain these skills. Athletes can optimize their movements, improve muscle memory, and develop more efficient techniques through neuroplasticity, leading to enhanced performance.

Mental resilience and adaptability: Neuroplasticity also contributes to an athlete's mental resilience and adaptability. By developing new cognitive strategies and emotional coping mechanisms, athletes can better handle setbacks, overcome performance anxiety, and maintain a positive outlook even in challenging situations. This mental resilience is essential for maintaining motivation, perseverance, and long-term success in sports.

Recovery from injury: In the event of an injury, neuroplasticity allows the brain to adapt and compensate for any physical limitations or changes. During recovery, the brain can reorganize its neural connections to help regain lost functions, develop new movement patterns, and facilitate rehabilitation. This adaptive capacity is crucial for athletes returning to their pre-injury performance levels.

The role of magic mushrooms in promoting neuroplasticity: Magic mushrooms, specifically their active compounds psilocybin and psilocin, have been shown to promote neuroplasticity. By stimulating the serotonin system, they can enhance learning, memory, and cognitive flexibility. This increased neuroplasticity may help athletes adapt more quickly to new training techniques, recover more efficiently from injuries, and develop mental resilience. However, it's essential to approach magic mushrooms with caution and a thorough understanding of their potential effects on the brain and athletic performance.

The impact of neuroplasticity on training and recovery highlights its significance in the world of athletics. By understanding and harnessing the power of neuroplasticity, athletes can optimize their performance, overcome challenges, and achieve their full potential.

Microdosing for Athletic Performance

Pursuing excellence in athletic endeavors often leads to innovations in training, nutrition, and mental techniques. Among these innovations, the art and science of microdosing has emerged as a notable frontier, promising to push the boundaries of what athletes believe is possible. While rooted in ancient traditions, this practice is finding its place in the modern performance optimization toolkit.

Microdosing, as the term suggests, operates on the principle of moderation. It is not about seeking the profound, transcendent experiences that one might associate with psychedelics, but rather about harnessing a consistent and measured dose to fine-tune the mind-body connection. Such delicate calibrations can, in the right context, lead to significant improvements in focus, resilience, and even physical endurance.

In the following pages, we will embark on a comprehensive journey, exploring the intricacies of microdosing and its implications for athletic prowess. We'll discuss its science, offering insights into how these diminutive doses interact with our physiology. We'll also guide you on crafting a microdosing strategy that aligns with your athletic aspirations, ensuring you're equipped with the knowledge to make informed decisions.

Moreover, by diving deep into firsthand accounts and meticulously researched case studies, this chapter offers a lens into the world of athletes who have dared to integrate this practice into their routines. Their stories, filled with challenges, successes, and illuminating insights, paint a comprehensive picture of microdosing's transformative potential in sports.

Understanding Microdosing: The Subtle Catalyst for Athletic Potential

Microdosing has emerged as a nuanced method of engaging with psychedelics. It's neither about seeking profound, hallucinogenic journeys nor entirely about medicinal benefits. Instead, it threads the needle, operating in a space where one can touch the fringe benefits of these powerful substances without veering off into the deep end of consciousness exploration. When we discuss taking 1/10th to 1/20th of a standard recreational dose of a substance like psilocybin, it's not to induce the kaleidoscopic visuals or deep introspective dives that psychedelics are known for. Instead, this fractional dosage subtly amplifies specific cognitive, emotional, and physical attributes.

The chemical dance that ensues when psilocybin mushrooms are consumed is both fascinating and intricate. As the body metabolizes psilocybin, it transforms into psilocin, its psychoactive relative, mingling with the brain's serotonin receptors.

This liaison, even at the sub-perceptual level of microdosing, can usher in enhanced well-being, clearer cognition, and a more fluid creative process. Think of it as a light switch being dimmed up just a notch, illuminating facets of one's mind and body that might have been slightly obscured.

For athletes, this illumination can be the difference between a routine training day and one where boundaries are pushed. After all, the realm of sports isn't just about raw physical prowess; it's an intricate blend of physicality, strategy, creativity, focus, and psychological endurance. Microdosing promises to be a tool in the athlete's kit, amplifying these attributes. Imagine the pinpoint focus required for a basketball player to take a free throw or the burst of creative strategy a soccer player needs to find a path through defenders. In these moments, the subtle enhancements of microdosing might be the nudge an athlete needs to perform at their peak.

Yet, it's crucial to understand microdosing's role in the grander scheme of athletic training. It isn't a miracle solution, nor does it replace the hours of dedicated training, nutritional balance, mental conditioning, and rest that athletes commit to. Instead, it complements these elements. When integrated judiciously into a comprehensive training regimen, microdosing becomes one of many tools to carve out the athlete's peak potential.

As this chapter unfolds, we'll further unpack the layers of microdosing, diving into the nuances that make it a compelling option for athletes. From its foundational science to real-world applications, we'll explore how this subtle psychedelic practice reshapes athletic performance's contours.

Enhanced Focus and Mental Clarity: The Cognitive Edge in Sports

In the high-stakes world of competitive sports, the minutiae matter. A slight increase in focus, an iota of better decision-making, or a flash of heightened perception can change the outcome of a game or race. Athletes increasingly use an unconventional method to glean these nuanced improvements: microdosing magic mushrooms.

Microdosing operates on the principle of utilizing minimal quantities of a substance to achieve specific, desired outcomes without venturing into more profound, altered states. For athletes, this could mean sharper reflexes during a tennis match, a more profound connection to their body's rhythm during a marathon, or even a more profound sense of calm before a significant competition.

Neurological Mechanism of Psilocybin:

The primary active ingredient in magic mushrooms, psilocybin, gets converted in the body to psilocin, which interacts with the brain's serotonin receptors. Serotonin, the 'feel good' neurotransmitter, plays crucial roles in mood regulation, sleep, appetite, and cognition. The augmentation of serotonin's action can lead to enhanced mood, sharper focus, and improved mental clarity. Additionally, evidence suggests that psychedelics can promote neurogenesis (the birth of new neurons) and enhance brain connectivity.

Practical Implications in Sports:
Enhanced focus can be pivotal in an athlete's performance. Imagine a sprinter maintaining a consistent stride rhythm, a basketball player making precise shots under pressure, or a gymnast executing a complex routine with absolute precision. A heightened mental clarity can allow an athlete to "be in the zone," that mental sweet spot where they're fully immersed and perform at their peak.

Day-to-Day Training Regimen:
Beyond competition, this enhanced focus is equally advantageous during daily training sessions. It can lead to better technique assimilation, effective feedback incorporation, and a more structured approach to training. As an athlete, understanding nuances and making micro-adjustments based on sensory feedback is crucial. The heightened state of awareness offered by microdosing is invaluable.

A Note on Variability:
It's crucial to note that individual responses to microdosing can vary. While many report enhanced clarity and focus, others might have yet to notice any significant changes. Dosing, body weight, metabolism, and genetic makeup can influence one's experience.

The Broader Perspective:

While the focus and clarity benefits of microdosing are enticing, they're just a facet of the broader picture. When woven into a holistic training approach that incorporates physical training, nutrition, rest, and mental conditioning, microdosing can amplify an athlete's journey to peak performance.

Incorporating microdosing into an athletic regimen is undoubtedly an intriguing frontier. However, athletes and coaches should approach it with an informed perspective, always prioritizing safety, ethics, and the spirit of the sport.

Benefits Unveiled: How Microdosing Elevates Athletic Prowess

As the athletic realm relentlessly pursues excellence, it often welcomes novel approaches to amplify performance. Recently, the interest in microdosing has burgeoned, presenting such an avenue. Athletes from diverse backgrounds are exploring its myriad potentialities, looking beyond the overtly psychedelic experience towards the nuanced effects of these sub-perceptual doses. These effects hold promise in uplifting numerous facets of athletic pursuits. As we delve into this topic, we aim to understand the multifaceted advantages athletes might harness through microdosing, providing insight into why this practice is rapidly gaining traction in athletic communities.

Cultivating Precision: In the realm of sports and athletic endeavors, the finest margins can often dictate the outcome of a competition. It's not merely about strength, speed, or endurance, but also the intricate nuances and details that can make all the difference. Precision, in this context, becomes paramount. Every move, every breath, and every decision has the potential to shift the balance of a game or race. This level of meticulous attention to detail differentiates good athletes from the greats.

Enter microdosing. This practice has been reported to elevate one's consciousness, amplifying focus and heightening awareness. Athletes, in these elevated states, can perceive and react to minute details that might be overlooked in a regular state.

For a gymnast, it might be the perfect alignment during a routine; for a sprinter, the exact moment to kick for the finish; and for a martial artist, the subtle shift in an opponent's stance signals their next move.

By enhancing their perception, athletes can train with a renewed level of precision, honing in on techniques and refining skills more accurately. The consistency and repetition in training, combined with the increased precision from microdosing, can lead to mastering complex maneuvers and techniques with a swiftness previously unattainable. In the ever-competitive world of sports, where every advantage counts, such precision can be the difference between victory and defeat.

Fueling Passion and Drive: An athlete's path is seldom a straight line; it is a winding road interspersed with moments of glory and bouts of challenges. Just as physical endurance is celebrated, the mental and emotional fortitude to persevere through setbacks is equally commendable. At times, even the most dedicated athletes can find their zeal waning, especially when faced with repeated obstacles or plateaus in their performance. In such moments, the distinction between those who merely participate and those who genuinely excel often comes down to sheer passion and drive.

Microdosing has emerged as a potential ally in this journey, bridging the athlete's current state and their untapped reservoirs of motivation. The subtle alterations in consciousness that it brings can foster a renewed sense of purpose. Rather than viewing challenges as insurmountable barriers, with the aid of microdosing, athletes might perceive them as opportunities for growth.

The introspective moments that microdosing can facilitate allow athletes to reconnect with the foundational reasons they chose their discipline in the first place. Rediscovering this core 'why' can be a profound source of renewed energy and determination. Whether it's the love of the game, the thrill of competition, or the personal satisfaction derived from self-improvement, these passions become more vivid, driving athletes to approach their training with a fresh zest.

The heightened emotional connectivity that some users report can further deepen the bond between an athlete and their discipline, making the daily grind of training a routine and deeply fulfilling pursuit. In essence, while physical skills and techniques are undeniably essential, it's the passion and drive that microdosing can amplify, which ensures that athletes stay engaged, inspired, and ever-ready to push the boundaries of what they believe possible.

Boosting Resilience and Stamina: The life of an athlete is a testament to the human body's incredible potential, but pushing those boundaries requires strength and recovery. Achieving peak performance is not just about the bursts of speed or power at the moment; it's also about how quickly one can bounce back, ready to do it all over again. This is where the intriguing potential of microdosing comes into play.

Stamina, in the athletic sense, extends beyond merely physical endurance—it encompasses the mental grit to persist even when the going gets tough. Many who have ventured into microdosing describe an enhanced sense of vitality, feeling like they've tapped into a dormant energy reserve. This can manifest as longer, more efficient training sessions or the ability to maintain focus and precision even in the later stages of a grueling competition. The clarity and alertness potentially fostered by microdosing can help an athlete tap into deeper reservoirs of endurance, making those extra miles or minutes seem more attainable.

Recovery is just as vital as the exertion itself. Anecdotal accounts from athletes who've integrated microdosing into their regimen often emphasize reduced recovery times. This is not just about healing physical wear and tear; it's also about mental and emotional rejuvenation. The aftermath of an intense competition or workout can sometimes leave one mentally drained, with a sense of inertia setting in. The subtle cognitive shifts from microdosing might pave the way for heightened neural plasticity, allowing the brain to recalibrate faster, and thus helping athletes to mentally "reset" more efficiently.

The potential anti-inflammatory properties of some psychedelics could theoretically play a role in this expedited recovery. While rigorous scientific data is still forthcoming, early research and anecdotal testimonies suggest that microdosing could help alleviate minor inflammations, reducing muscle soreness and hastening the body's natural healing process.

In the dynamic, demanding realm of sports, where athletes are perpetually seeking ways to edge past their competitors and their personal bests, the dual boon of increased stamina and quicker recovery offered by microdosing could be a game-changer. However, it's essential to approach this with a discerning mind, understanding that individual responses may vary, and more comprehensive studies are needed to validate these claims fully.

Navigating Performance Pressures: The athletic world is a crucible of pressure, where the intensity of competition often reaches feverish heights. The demands can be immense, and not just from the perspective of physical prowess; the psychological burden is equally taxing. Expectations from coaches, fans, sponsors, and even oneself can create a vortex of stress that is both relentless and all-encompassing. How one responds to these pressures can define a career, turning potential champions into legends or, conversely, undermining even the most gifted athletes. In this complex emotional landscape, microdosing might offer an intriguing pathway, enabling athletes to navigate these pressures with grace, composure, and poise.

Microdosing fosters a serene and centered mindset, potentially mitigating anxiety and heightening emotional intelligence. Unlike higher doses of psychedelics, which can induce profound perceptual shifts, the sub-perceptual nature of microdosing is often described as a gentle tuning of one's emotional and cognitive receptors. This can translate into increased mindfulness, an enhanced connection with the present moment, and a more nuanced understanding of one's emotional landscape.

Such mental alignment might aid an athlete in deciphering the underlying sources of stress and pressure, transforming these hindrances into motivational fuel rather than debilitating obstacles. The ability to remain grounded, even in the whirlwind of a high-stakes competition, can be the difference between victory and defeat. By promoting inner harmony and resilience, microdosing may help athletes approach their craft with a tranquility that is both self-assured and adaptive.

This state of equilibrium could lead to more effective communication with teammates, coaches, and support staff. In sports where collaboration and synergy are essential, the enhanced empathy and openness that microdosing might foster could pave the way for a more harmonious and efficient team dynamic.

However, it's crucial to recognize that microdosing is not a panacea. While it may offer unique insights and coping mechanisms, its success likely relies on integration within a broader psychological and physical support framework. Proper guidance, informed decisions, responsible use, and a thorough understanding of the potential benefits and the existing legal framework must be the cornerstone of any such endeavor.

As more athletes share their experiences and scientific research gradually unfolds the layers of understanding, microdosing's role in navigating performance pressures could evolve from anecdotal curiosity to a studied component of modern athletic training. But for now, it remains an intriguing possibility, beckoning athletes who seek a novel way to approach the mental rigors of their demanding profession.

Fostering Symbiotic Harmony: In the dynamic world of sports, where split-second decisions can be the difference between triumph and defeat, the synergy between mind and body isn't just an advantage—it's an essential component of excellence. The connection between mental cognition and physical execution defines athletes' ability to perform at the highest levels, allowing them to respond intuitively to challenges and adapt their strategies in real-time. Microdosing is emerging as a unique practice that might facilitate and deepen this essential connection, letting athletes tune into their body's cues with enhanced sensitivity and acuity.

The athlete's ability to perceive, interpret, and respond to sensory information is at the heart of the symbiotic harmony between mind and body. Whether it's the tactile feedback from a tennis racket, the auditory cues in a team sport, or the proprioceptive sense of balance in gymnastics, an athlete's senses are their immediate link to the physical world. Microdosing has been reported to enhance sensory perception, possibly leading to a more detailed awareness of one's body in space and time. This heightened sensory engagement can translate into more precise movements, greater coordination, and an intuitive understanding of physical dynamics.

The mental aspect of athletic performance often revolves around focus, presence, and the ability to stay grounded in the moment.

Whether internal or external, distractions can disrupt this focus, leading to mistakes and missed opportunities. Microdosing may cultivate a deeper state of mindfulness, helping athletes remain centered and fully engaged with the task. They can respond to changes and challenges with fluidity and grace by fostering a greater connection to the present moment.

An athlete's journey is one of constant growth, adaptation, and learning. Understanding one's body, recognizing its strengths and weaknesses, and adapting training strategies accordingly is pivotal for progress. The enhanced mind-body connection fostered by microdosing facilitates this learning process. Athletes are more attuned to subtle feedback, more receptive to corrections, and more intuitive in adjusting their techniques. This can lead to more efficient training, faster skill acquisition, and a more personalized approach to their discipline.

Beyond the immediate realm of performance, the synergistic alignment between mind and body plays a significant role in an athlete's overall well-being. The balance, integration, and understanding of physical and mental health can be critical in preventing injuries, managing stress, and ensuring a sustainable and fulfilling athletic career. Microdosing might contribute to this holistic understanding, helping athletes maintain this balance with increased awareness and care.

The potential of microdosing in fostering symbiotic harmony likely doesn't exist in isolation. Integrating it with other mindfulness practices, physical therapies, and mental training techniques could enhance its efficacy. Coordination with coaches, healthcare professionals, and sports psychologists may ensure that the practice aligns with the athlete's overall training strategy and complies with legal and ethical considerations.

The exploration of microdosing in fostering mind-body harmony is still in its infancy, and the landscape is filled with promise and uncertainty. Further research, responsible experimentation, and an open dialogue within the athletic community will be essential in understanding and harnessing this complex and nuanced relationship. But the preliminary insights and anecdotal accounts offer an intriguing glimpse into a frontier that could reshape how athletes connect with their bodies and their sport.

Mastering Concentration: Concentration is paramount in sports, where even a fleeting distraction can result in defeat. Microdosing has been associated with a heightened ability to concentrate, enabling athletes to remain steadfastly focused on their tasks, whether in a rigorous training session or a critical competitive event.

The concept of concentration in athletics extends far beyond simple attention to detail. It encompasses an athlete's ability to fully immerse themselves in the present moment, shutting out irrelevant stimuli and focusing solely on the task. This hyper-focused state can lead to what athletes often describe as "being in the zone" – a state of optimal performance where actions flow seamlessly and intuitively. Microdosing might contribute to this state by sharpening mental clarity and enhancing an athlete's ability to focus on the present moment.

This mastery of focus can have tangible effects on performance. In disciplines that require extreme precision, such as archery, golf, or shooting, even the slightest distraction can have significant consequences. Microdosing may fine-tune the mind's ability to zero in on a specific target, eliminate peripheral distractions, and execute movements with meticulous accuracy.

In team sports, where rapid decision-making and coordination with teammates are essential, sustaining concentration enables athletes to process information quickly and respond appropriately. An enhanced focus could lead to better understanding and prediction of teammates' movements, more effective communication, and a smoother flow in executing team strategies.

The benefits of concentration extend to training as well. Consistency, effort, and the meticulous repetition of specific skills are foundational to athletic development. Microdosing might aid in maintaining the mental stamina needed to endure long and intensive training sessions, promoting a state of concentration that allows athletes to absorb technical corrections, refine their skills, and develop new strategies without fatigue or waning interest.

Yet, it's essential to recognize that concentration isn't merely a solitary endeavor. Athletes must also be able to switch focus rapidly, from narrow to broad and from internal to external, adapting to the ever-changing competition dynamics. Microdosing might aid in sharpening focus and enhancing cognitive flexibility, allowing athletes to shift their attention as required, adjusting to the ebbs and flows of competition.

Of course, mastering concentration through microdosing has its complexities. Legal and ethical considerations, individual variations in response, and the need for guidance and supervision make this a nuanced subject. Additionally, this potential benefit of microdosing should not be viewed as a standalone solution but as part of a broader strategy to improve mental skills, possibly complementing other concentration-enhancing practices like meditation or cognitive training.

The relationship between microdosing and concentration in sports offers an exciting frontier with promising possibilities. As researchers delve further into this area and more athletes share their experiences, the nuanced ways microdosing may contribute to the mastery of focus will likely continue to unfold. For now, it remains an intriguing tool, with potential applications ranging from skill development and performance enhancement to the deeper mental well-being of athletes.

Uplifting the Spirit: The world of athletics calls for physical prowess, relentless enthusiasm, and love for the sport. Athletes often face a mental battle to keep their passion alive, especially during intense training, recovery from injury, or unexpected setbacks. A growing consensus among users and some research indicate that microdosing may play a role in uplifting the mood, thereby rekindling an athlete's intrinsic motivation and zeal for their chosen discipline.

This uplifting of spirit is not merely about feeling happy or content. It's about a deeper connection to the sport, a resurgence of passion, and a renewed commitment to pursuing excellence. Microdosing might spark this by subtly shifting an athlete's perspective, helping them reconnect with the joy and fulfillment initially drew them to their sport. This can be particularly beneficial during challenging times when motivation might wane.

Maintaining a positive and enthusiastic mindset becomes critical in the competitive landscape of athletics, where external pressures and expectations can be overwhelming. Microdosing might foster a sense of resilience, enabling athletes to focus on the positives and stay inspired despite their adversities.

This uplifted state of mind may translate into tangible performance benefits. A positive mood often leads to increased energy levels, greater creativity in problem-solving, and more fluidity in physical movements. For example, an invigorated athlete may approach training with renewed vigor, experiment with novel strategies, and recover more rapidly from physical exertion.

The upbeat mood induced by microdosing might enhance an athlete's relationship with coaches, teammates, and support staff. A more positive, engaged, and motivated athlete may contribute to a more cohesive team environment, leading to collective success.

However, it's vital to approach this potential benefit with caution and awareness. The relationship between mood and performance is complex, and microdosing is not a one-size-fits-all solution. Factors such as individual personality, the nature of the sport, the specific substance used for microdosing, and the context in which it is done all play a role in determining its effectiveness in uplifting the spirit.

While microdosing may be beneficial in enhancing mood, it is not a replacement for sound mental health practices, professional psychological support, or a well-rounded approach to maintaining enthusiasm for the sport. Proper guidance, ethical considerations, and an understanding of the broader context are essential when considering microdosing to enhance mood in athletics.

The potential of microdosing to uplift the spirit of athletes offers an intriguing possibility within the context of modern sports psychology. While promising, it is a field that requires further exploration, scientific investigation, and ethical consideration. As part of a comprehensive approach to mental well-being and performance enhancement, microdosing might serve as a valuable adjunct, helping athletes rediscover their passion, enhance their resilience, and thrive in their pursuit of athletic excellence.

Strengthening Stamina and Prompt Recovery: The challenges of prolonged athletic activity and the necessity for swift recovery lie at the core of any athletic pursuit. In this intricate dance of physical demand and resilience, microdosing has emerged as a potential tool for some athletes. Those who have experimented with this practice have observed enhanced endurance during grueling workouts and quicker recovery afterward. Unlike a sudden burst of energy, this subtle increase in stamina allows athletes to push their boundaries without immediate exhaustion.

The enhancement in endurance may also be connected to a mental shift that allows athletes to maximize their performance by immersing themselves wholly in their training. The subtle increase in stamina promotes a more sustained and focused effort, leading to potentially higher productivity in practice and improved outcomes in competition.

Alongside this boost in stamina, there are hints at microdosing's potential in aiding faster physical recovery. This might involve reduced muscle soreness or enhanced cellular repair, preparing athletes for their next challenge more quickly. The recuperative effects extend to mental recovery, assisting athletes in returning to mental equilibrium more quickly after a demanding workout or competition.

However, it's essential to recognize that these benefits are not universal and may vary based on individual factors, sport type, and the substance used. Moreover, while these benefits appear promising, they are often based on personal testimonies and limited studies, so more rigorous research is needed.

The potential to strengthen stamina and promote prompt recovery through microdosing is tantalizing. If pursued, it should be considered part of a broader, holistic approach to training, stamina building, and recovery, not a standalone solution. It requires careful consideration, a personalized approach, and, ideally, professional guidance.

Whether or not microdosing can truly revolutionize these aspects of athletic performance remains a question that awaits further exploration and scientific validation. The potential implications of these findings extend far beyond individual athletes and have the power to influence coaching methodologies, training paradigms, and even the broader philosophy of sport and performance enhancement.

Managing the Mental Game: High-stakes competitions come with their share of anxiety and stress, which can be overwhelming even for seasoned athletes. In these intense moments, microdosing is emerging as a valuable asset, helping athletes maintain a composed demeanor, which is vital for strategic thinking and decision-making during crunch moments.

The anxiolytic effects of microdosing create a sense of calm and focus that transcends the traditional boundaries of athletic training. This tranquility enables athletes to stay centered, approach challenges strategically, and make quick, accurate decisions in pressure-cooker situations. Whether in a championship game or a local competition, the ability to remain calm and collected can be the difference between victory and defeat.

This mental composure is not confined to competition day alone but extends to the rigorous training periods leading up to it. Preparation for significant events requires intense concentration, resilience, and the ability to cope with the weight of expectations. Through microdosing, athletes may find a tool that supports a positive and focused mindset throughout the preparatory phase, turning potential stressors into sources of motivation and inspiration.

Microdosing also complements other psychological tools and techniques, such as meditation, visualization, and professional mental coaching. By integrating it into a holistic mental wellness strategy, athletes can forge a mental edge that stands up to the most demanding competitive environments.

In sports where the margin for error is minimal, and the mental game is often as crucial as physical prowess, microdosing opens new horizons for performance enhancement. The synergy between the mind and the substance in maintaining composure, enhancing focus, and strategic decision-making has positioned microdosing as an exciting avenue within athletic performance optimization.

The application of microdosing in managing the mental aspects of athletic performance represents a groundbreaking approach. By fostering a sense of balance and tranquility in the high-pressure world of competitive sports, microdosing can revolutionize how athletes prepare and perform, taking them one step closer to their ultimate goals. This exploration into the mind's potential underscores the complexity and beauty of human performance, and microdosing stands as a promising piece in the intricate puzzle of athletic excellence.

Deepening the Mind-Body Synergy: The harmonious relationship between the mind and body is a cornerstone of success in athletic performance. The ability to interpret the body's subtle signals, adapt to its needs, and respond with appropriate actions is a skill that often distinguishes top-performing athletes. Microdosing offers a way to sharpen this mind-body dialogue, enhancing an athlete's ability to intuitively gauge their body's needs, whether it's rest, nutrition, or specific training modalities.

This heightened awareness goes beyond merely avoiding injury or fatigue; it empowers athletes to connect with their physical selves more profoundly. By doing so, they can tap into a reservoir of insights into how their body reacts to different training techniques, nutritional adjustments, or recovery strategies. This nuanced understanding of one's body can lead to tailored training regimens that cater to an individual's unique physiological makeup.

Through microdosing, athletes may also discover an enhanced kinesthetic sense and a heightened awareness of their body's position and movement. This improvement can translate into more precise control and coordination, enabling more efficient movement and technique refinement. In disciplines where fine motor control and spatial awareness are crucial, such as gymnastics or ballet, this increased sensitivity to body movement can be an invaluable asset.

Integrating microdosing into an athlete's routine represents an ongoing dialogue with one's body. It is a continuous learning, adapting, and growing process that extends well beyond the training ground. By recognizing the signs that the body provides, athletes can optimize every aspect of their routine, from sleep and nutrition to training intensity and recovery strategies.

The mind-body synergy fostered through microdosing can also enrich the emotional and spiritual connection to the sport. The enhanced sensitivity and receptiveness may lead to a more profound appreciation of the beauty and grace inherent in the athletic pursuit, elevating the experience from mere physical exertion to an art form.

The role of microdosing in deepening the mind-body synergy illustrates its multifaceted potential within the athletic domain. By unlocking a more intimate understanding of one's physicality and aligning training strategies with intrinsic needs, athletes can create a more harmonious, effective, and fulfilling practice. This symbiosis between body and mind reflects the holistic nature of sports. It is a testament to the extraordinary potential of integrating microdosing into athletics. The era of personalized, intuitive training is upon us, and microdosing is an exciting tool in this new frontier of human performance.

Addressing Physical Discomforts: Athletic training, particularly at a competitive level, often involves pushing the body to its limits. This strenuous pursuit of excellence can sometimes lead to aches, soreness, and minor injuries that hinder consistent training and performance. Some athletes have found that microdosing offers a unique way to alleviate certain physical discomforts, allowing them to maintain their training regimen without being sidelined by these minor setbacks.

Solving physical discomfort through microdosing is not merely about masking pain but fostering a more in-depth understanding of the body's needs. By enhancing the body's feedback mechanisms, microdosing allows athletes to discern better the difference between a severe injury that requires rest and minor discomfort that can be worked through. This nuanced perception can guide athletes in modifying their training techniques, introducing targeted stretches, or adapting their recovery practices, thus preventing further discomfort or injury.

In addition to this intuitive awareness, microdosing may provide direct physical benefits contributing to comfort and recovery. For example, some athletes report a reduction in inflammation and muscle tension. This relief can be vital during intensive training periods or in sports that demand repetitive motions, where persistent discomfort can disrupt focus and lead to compensatory movement patterns that are less efficient or harmful.

The connection between the mind and body fostered through microdosing also enhances an athlete's ability to employ visualization techniques, a well-established practice in sports psychology. By vividly imagining the proper execution of a movement, athletes can align their bodies more accurately with their mental blueprint. Microdosing may intensify this connection, allowing athletes to visualize more clearly and translate these mental rehearsals more effectively into physical performance.

The potential of microdosing to elevate mood and reduce anxiety can contribute to a more positive relationship with training, even in the face of physical discomfort. Maintaining a positive outlook and staying committed to training, despite minor aches and pains, is crucial for long-term success. By promoting a balanced mental state, microdosing can help athletes persevere through the inevitable challenges of their athletic journey.

Microdosing can be a supportive tool in managing the physical discomforts often associated with rigorous training. By sharpening the athlete's awareness of their body's signals and potentially offering direct relief from inflammation and tension, microdosing can become an integral part of a comprehensive training and recovery strategy. As athletes continue to explore the benefits of this practice, the dialogue around microdosing is poised to grow, contributing to a broader understanding of holistic health and performance optimization in sports. The potential of microdosing to transform how athletes train, recover, and perform is a compelling testament to its emerging role in modern athletic endeavors.

Enhancing Sensory Perception: A keen sense of perception can translate into split-second advantages that distinguish triumph and defeat in sports. Every sport requires athletes to process sensory information, including sight, sound, touch, and proprioception (the sense of body position). Heightened sensory perception enables athletes to react faster, move more precisely, and maintain greater awareness of their surroundings, all essential for optimal performance. Microdosing, potentially enhancing these sensory faculties, is increasingly seen as a valuable tool in the athlete's arsenal.

Whether it's a tennis player reacting to the spin of an incoming serve, a soccer goalkeeper anticipating the trajectory of a penalty kick, or a runner sensing the texture of the ground beneath their feet, athletes continuously rely on sensory input to make decisions. This sensory information, when processed quickly and accurately, informs everything from strategic planning to physical response.

Microdosing's potential to heighten sensory perception stems from its effect on cognitive processing. Increasing neural connectivity and promoting a more fluid exchange of information within the brain, microdosing may allow athletes to process sensory input more efficiently. This can translate into a more nuanced understanding of their environment and an enhanced ability to respond to it.

For instance, in sports like basketball or football, a player's ability to hear the subtle sounds of opposing players' movements can give them an edge in anticipating plays. A boxer might sharpen their vision to detect the subtle shifts in an opponent's stance that signal an incoming punch. In endurance sports like cycling or long-distance running, the ability to feel subtle changes in terrain can guide pacing and prevent missteps.

The potential of microdosing to deepen sensory perception is about amplifying individual senses and integrating them into a more coherent and holistic understanding of the athletic context. This integration allows athletes to make more informed decisions during performance. For example, a baseball player who can simultaneously track the ball's flight, hear the coach's instructions, and feel the exact positioning of their body can coordinate these inputs to execute a perfect catch.

This enhancement of sensory perception can also contribute to more effective training. By becoming more attuned to the body's signals and subtle environmental cues, athletes can refine their techniques, develop better timing, and build a more instinctive and fluid relationship with their sport.

It is worth noting that enhancing sensory perception through microdosing is not about creating superhuman senses but rather about fine-tuning what is already present. It's about nurturing a more attentive and conscious engagement with the athletic experience, amplifying the nuanced dance between mind and body, and the dynamic interplay with the surrounding environment.

The potential of microdosing to enhance sensory perception represents a fascinating frontier in sports performance. By fostering a more attuned and integrated sensory experience, microdosing may help athletes reach new heights of responsiveness and adaptability. As more athletes explore this practice and share their insights, understanding how microdosing can contribute to heightened sensory perception will continue to evolve, potentially redefining how we approach training and competition in sports.

While these benefits offer a compelling case for microdosing in athletics, individual responses can vary widely. It's essential to approach this practice with a well-informed perspective, keeping abreast of the latest research and always prioritizing one's health and well-being.

Developing a Microdosing Protocol for Athletic Training

Creating a personalized microdosing protocol for athletic training involves several factors to ensure optimal results and safety. Here are some critical steps to consider when developing your own microdosing protocol for athletic performance enhancement:

Determine your dosage: Start with a low dose of psilocybin, typically between 0.1 to 0.3 grams of dried magic mushrooms or the equivalent in psilocybin extract. The goal is to find a dosage that provides subtle benefits without causing noticeable psychedelic effects. Remember that individual responses to microdosing may vary, so it's crucial to find the correct dose for you.

Establish a dosing schedule: Consistency is essential when microdosing for athletic performance. Many athletes follow a schedule of dosing every third day (one day on, two days off) to prevent developing a tolerance to psilocybin. However, you can adjust the frequency based on your needs and how your body responds to the substance. Make sure to track your dosing schedule and any effects you experience in a journal to better understand how microdosing affects your performance.

Monitor your physical and mental well-being: While microdosing, pay close attention to your physical and mental state. Track any mood, energy, focus, or recovery changes, and adjust your dosage or schedule accordingly. It's important to remember that microdosing is not a one-size-fits-all approach, and you may need to experiment with different dosages and schedules to find the optimal balance for your unique needs.

Combine microdosing with other performance-enhancing strategies: For the best results, incorporate microdosing into a holistic athletic training plan that includes proper nutrition, sleep, hydration, and mindfulness practices. This comprehensive approach will help you maximize the potential benefits of microdosing while supporting your overall health and well-being.

Prioritize safety: As with any substance, it's crucial to prioritize safety when microdosing for athletic performance. Always source your magic mushrooms or psilocybin extract from a reputable supplier to ensure purity and quality. If you're taking any medications or have pre-existing medical conditions, consult with a healthcare professional before beginning a microdosing regimen. Additionally, be mindful of the legal status of magic mushrooms in your location.

Following these steps, you can develop a personalized microdosing protocol that supports your athletic performance goals and helps you reach your full potential. Remember that patience and self-awareness are essential during this process, as it may take some time to fine-tune the ideal microdosing regimen for your specific needs.

Real-life Examples and Case Studies

In this section, we will explore a few real-life examples and case studies of athletes who have incorporated microdosing into their training regimen and experienced significant improvements in their performance.

A competitive cyclist, James began microdosing psilocybin to enhance his focus and endurance on long rides. After experimenting with different dosages, he found that taking 0.2 grams of dried magic mushrooms every third day significantly improved his mental clarity and allowed him to maintain a higher energy level throughout his training sessions. As a result, James saw improvements in his race times and overall performance.

Sarah, a professional weightlifter, started microdosing to help her cope with the mental challenges of her sport. By taking 0.15 grams of dried magic mushrooms on a one-day on, two days off schedule, she noticed increased motivation, mental resilience, and ability to push through challenging training sessions. Over time, Sarah's performance improved over time, and she attributed these gains partly to her microdosing protocol.

Mike, a marathon runner, turned to microdosing to aid his recovery and manage the physical demands of his training. After incorporating a regimen of 0.25 grams of dried magic mushrooms every fourth day, he reported experiencing less muscle soreness and faster recovery times, allowing him to maintain a more rigorous training schedule.

Laura, a professional dancer, started microdosing to enhance her mind-body connection and improve her creativity in choreography. Taking 0.1 grams of dried magic mushrooms every third day, Laura experienced increased focus and a deeper connection to her body, which allowed her to express herself more freely and innovate in her performances.

Emma, a professional soccer player, began microdosing to help her manage stress and anxiety related to high-pressure games and competitions. By taking 0.15 grams of dried magic mushrooms every third day, she noticed a significant reduction in her anxiety levels, leading to improved decision-making and performance on the field.

Alex, a mixed martial artist, incorporated microdosing into his training to enhance his mental flexibility and adaptability during fights. Using 0.2 grams of dried magic mushrooms every fourth day, he found that his ability to quickly strategize and respond to his opponent's moves improved, giving him a competitive edge in the ring.

A professional rock climber, Natalie started microdosing to increase her focus and mental stamina during long, challenging climbs. By taking 0.25 grams of dried magic mushrooms every three days, she reported enhanced concentration, better problem-solving abilities, and increased calm and confidence while climbing.

Richard, an Olympic swimmer, began microdosing to help him cope with the pressure of high-stakes competitions and improve his mental resilience. Using 0.1 grams of dried magic mushrooms on a one-day on, two days off schedule, he found that his pre-race anxiety decreased, and he was better able to maintain a positive mindset throughout his races, leading to improved performance and personal records.

Sarah, a long-distance runner, started microdosing to help her push through mental barriers and increase her endurance during marathon training. By taking 0.2 grams of dried magic mushrooms every four days, she discovered that her mental stamina improved, and she could maintain a consistent pace during her long runs without experiencing mental fatigue.

Michael, a professional cyclist, began microdosing to enhance his focus and reduce distractions during races. With a microdosing schedule of 0.15 grams of dried magic mushrooms every third day, he noticed improved concentration, a heightened sense of presence, and better overall race performance.

A competitive weightlifter, Vanessa incorporated microdosing into her training routine to improve her mind-muscle connection and enhance her proprioception. Taking 0.1 grams of dried magic mushrooms every three days, she reported a heightened awareness of her body's movements, leading to more efficient and powerful lifts.

A semiprofessional basketball player, Ethan started microdosing to cultivate better teamwork and communication skills on the court. Using 0.25 grams of dried magic mushrooms every fourth day, he found that his ability to read his teammates' movements and coordinate plays improved significantly, resulting in better team performance during games.

These examples illustrate the potential benefits of microdosing for athletes across various disciplines. It's essential to remember that individual responses to microdosing may vary, and what works for one person may not necessarily work for another. By carefully experimenting with different dosages and schedules, and incorporating microdosing into a comprehensive training plan, athletes can unlock new levels of performance and personal growth.

Macrodosing for Transformative Breakthroughs

In this chapter, we delve into the world of macrodosing magic mushrooms and their potential to facilitate transformative breakthroughs that can benefit athletes both personally and professionally. Macrodosing refers to taking larger doses of magic mushrooms, typically 2-5 grams of dried material, to induce a psychedelic experience. While microdosing aims to enhance physical and mental performance subtly, macrodosing can lead to profound shifts in self-awareness, personal growth, and overall well-being.

We will explore the power of macrodosing to help athletes overcome mental blocks, fears, and limiting beliefs that may be holding them back from reaching their full potential. We will also discuss the importance of enhancing the mind-body connection to optimize performance and create a supportive setting for macrodosing sessions. Additionally, we will share personal experiences and case studies to demonstrate the potential impact of macrodosing on athletic performance and personal growth.

As athletes venture into macrodosing, it's crucial to approach these experiences with an open mind, respect for the substance, and an understanding of the potential challenges and breakthroughs that may arise. By embracing the insights and lessons gained through macrodosing, athletes can unlock new levels of performance, resilience, and self-awareness.

The Power of Macrodosing for Personal Growth

In contrast to microdosing's subtle shifts in cognition, macrodosing, or the ingestion of more significant amounts of psychedelic substances like magic mushrooms, offers a profound and transformative journey. This journey can be instrumental in personal growth and self-discovery, and its implications for athletes are noteworthy and multifaceted.

Understanding the Self and Breaking Barriers: Macrodosing is a gateway to deep introspection, taking the individual on an immersive journey into the self. For athletes, the experience often manifests in startling revelations illuminating previously unrecognized self-imposed limitations, fears, and deeply rooted patterns. These inhibitions may have silently obstructed personal growth and athletic achievement for years.

Unearthing these barriers is akin to exposing hidden fractures in the foundation of one's psyche. It's not merely an intellectual understanding; it's a visceral encounter with the constraints that have shaped an athlete's mental landscape. It's a confrontation with the self, facilitated by the profound clarity that macrodosing can bring.

Realization is only the first step in a transformative process. The real power of macrodosing lies in its capacity to assist athletes in dismantling these discovered barriers. By confronting them with a courage born of clear-sightedness, individuals can begin to chip away at the walls that have contained them. Whether it's a fear of failure, a limiting belief about one's abilities, or a harmful pattern of self-criticism, macrodosing offers a space to challenge and overcome these obstacles.

What follows the confrontation is often a cathartic release and a paving of the path towards higher levels of achievement. The intense emotional outpouring that accompanies the tearing down of these internal walls can be both healing and empowering. It allows for the emergence of newfound confidence and courage that extends beyond the athletic field into all facets of life.

The macrodosing experience often culminates in the reshaping of personal narratives. The insights gained lead to a reframing of one's self-story, breaking free from stifling mindsets and limited perspectives. It allows athletes to author a new narrative that is not confined by past fears or patterns but driven by empowerment, ambition, and a revitalized sense of purpose.

Macrodosing can be a key that unlocks profound personal growth for athletes. By delving into the hidden recesses of the mind, uncovering and confronting what lies beneath, it provides a pathway to transcend old limitations. It's a process that involves understanding, confrontation, release, and reconstruction, all aimed at forging a stronger, more resilient self. For those in the relentless pursuit of excellence, it can be an invaluable tool, opening doors to levels of performance and personal fulfillment that might have previously seemed unattainable.

Cultivating Mental Resilience: The world of sports is fraught with relentless challenges, adversities, and pressures. Pursuing excellence requires an unyielding mental fortitude to weather the storms of failure, setbacks, and grueling competition. Macrodosing, with its profound and often intense psychedelic experiences, emerges as an unconventional yet potent tool for fostering this essential resilience.

During a macrodosing session, the mind's landscape transforms into a terrain of intricate emotional and cognitive vistas. These are not mere abstract thoughts or fleeting emotions; they are palpable, immersive experiences that can take various shapes. For some, it might be a confrontation with deep-seated fears or past traumas. For others, it could be an intense grappling with existential questions and personal values. The terrain is as varied as the individuals who traverse it.

The path through these inner landscapes can be arduous, requiring the individual to face and navigate challenges that may be both startling and complex. It's akin to an inner odyssey, where the trials and tribulations symbolize the broader struggles in one's life, including those within the athletic realm.

As athletes embark on this inner journey, facing these mental and emotional landscapes is a training ground for resilience. It's a space where they can learn to endure, persevere, and emerge stronger. Each challenge faced and overcome within the psychedelic experience translates into inner strength that can be carried forward into their athletic pursuits.

The macrodosing experience, therefore, acts as a crucible for mental fortitude. By traversing challenging terrains within the mind, athletes are, in essence, rehearsing for the real-world challenges they face on the playing field. The determination, courage, and unshakeable resolve cultivated during a macrodosing session become transferable skills. They are tools that can be wielded during training, in competitions, and in the face of setbacks and failures.

The insights gained from facing inner challenges can lead to a greater understanding of oneself, enhancing mental clarity and focus. This clear-headed determination can be instrumental in maintaining a steely focus on goals, irrespective of external pressures or distractions.

The practice of macrodosing is more than just an exploration of consciousness; it's a strategic endeavor to build mental resilience. For athletes, this inner strength, once honed and refined, becomes a robust armor, empowering them to persevere and triumph over the adversities, setbacks, and intense pressures inherent in competitive sports. With its trials and triumphs, the psychedelic journey becomes a metaphorical arena where athletes can develop the unbreakable resolve needed to excel in their chosen field. It adds a profound layer to their training, transcending physical conditioning, and fostering a resilient mind that stands unshaken in the face of challenges.

Aligning Goals and Values: In the intense world of competitive sports, aligning goals with deeper personal values is not just a philosophical consideration; it's a tangible factor that can markedly influence an athlete's performance and fulfillment. This alignment forms the core of what motivates an athlete, steering their passion, driving their commitment, and defining the very essence of their sporting journey. Macrodosing, with its potential to prompt profound introspection and self-discovery, catalyzes this alignment process, unlocking levels of intrinsic motivation and purpose that can elevate an athlete's pursuit from mere competition to a deeply meaningful quest.

The macrodosing experience often immerses an individual in a contemplative space where the ordinary barriers of ego and superficial thinking are transcended. This allows a deep exploration into the core values, beliefs, and existential concerns that shape a person's identity. For athletes, this exploration is an opportunity to understand what truly drives them, whether it's the love for the sport, the desire to excel, or a commitment to a greater cause. These answers can define the very soul of their athletic journey.

Once these core values are unearthed, the next step is aligning them with sporting goals. This means connecting the personal values discovered during the macrodosing experience with the athlete's ambitions, strategies, and daily routines in their sport. This alignment is not merely intellectual; it's visceral and deeply emotional. It's about infusing the daily grind of training, the thrill of competition, and the inevitable setbacks with a profound sense of purpose that resonates with the athlete's inner self.

The alignment of values and goals is not static; it's dynamic and continually evolving. It transforms the pursuit of sporting excellence into something far more significant. It becomes a quest, a profoundly personal journey imbued with passion, purpose, and a connection to something transcendent. This connection can range from personal growth and self-mastery to a commitment to community, spiritual, or philosophical ideology.

With this alignment, the sporting pursuit ceases to be merely about winning or losing. It evolves into a narrative where every training session, every competition, and every failure or success becomes a chapter in a grander story. It's a story where the sport becomes a vehicle for personal growth, self-expression, and realizing a greater vision.

This profound connection between values and goals can become a wellspring of intrinsic motivation. It fuels the athlete's drive not from external rewards or recognition but from an inner compulsion aligned with their true self. This intrinsic motivation is often more sustainable, resilient to failures, and fulfilling in the long run.

In essence, macrodosing offers athletes a unique pathway to delve into their innermost selves, uncovering values and motivations that may have been obscured or neglected. The practice can transform the sporting journey into a profound personal quest by facilitating this deep alignment between personal values and athletic goals. It's an alchemy that transcends the superficialities of competition, instilling a sense of meaning, passion, and purpose that can enhance performance and the overall quality of the athletic experience. The result is a harmonious fusion of sport with self, where every sprint, every leap, every triumph, and every defeat is part of a grand tapestry woven with the threads of the athlete's most profound beliefs and desires.

Enhancing Creativity and Adaptability: The rigorous demands of athletic competition often require more than just physical prowess and technical mastery. Creativity, adaptability, and innovation can be key differentiators, setting champions apart. Sports are dynamic and ever-changing, with situations and challenges that can turn in unexpected directions at any moment.

The agility to adapt, the creativity to devise novel strategies, and the flexibility to change course as the situation demands can give athletes a competitive edge. Macrodosing, with its capacity to enhance these cognitive qualities, has emerged as a fascinating avenue to explore these possibilities.

Unlocking creative potential is one of the robust attributes that macrodosing may foster in athletes. In psychedelics, macrodosing has been linked to significant increases in creativity. By altering typical thinking patterns and opening the mind to new pathways of thought, a psychedelic journey can dissolve mental barriers and unleash a torrent of creative energy. For athletes, this creativity is not just about artistic expression; it's about finding novel ways to approach their sport, devising innovative techniques, and seeing opportunities where others might see obstacles. Whether it's a soccer player finding an unexpected angle for a pass, a basketball player executing an unconventional play, or a martial artist applying an unorthodox technique, creativity can manifest in countless ways across various sports.

The complex landscape of sports often presents problems that need rapid solutions. Enhancing problem-solving skills through macrodosing can be vital to an athlete's toolkit. A sudden change in weather during an outdoor competition, an unexpected injury, or a shift in the opponent's strategy can all demand quick and effective problem-solving. Macrodosing has been associated with enhanced lateral thinking and seeing problems from different angles. This can equip athletes with the skills to navigate these challenges quickly and confidently, turning potential setbacks into opportunities for success.

Fostering flexibility in thought patterns is another area where macrodosing may contribute significantly. Rigid thinking can be a limitation in sports, where adaptability often reigns supreme. The macrodosing experience has been found to promote flexibility in thought patterns that allow for more fluid thinking.

This adaptability can be a valuable asset for athletes, allowing them to adjust their strategies, react to unexpected developments with poise, and remain open to new ways of approaching their sport. This mental agility translates into performance, enabling athletes to stay ahead of the game, regardless of what comes their way.

Infusing the game with fresh perspectives through macrodosing can also breathe new life into an athlete's approach to their sport. Sometimes, an athlete's growth and improvement can be hindered by stale routines and entrenched ways of thinking. By reshuffling cognitive frameworks and offering fresh perspectives, macrodosing can lead to a rejuvenated passion for the sport, an openness to new techniques, and a willingness to take calculated risks that might lead to breakthrough performances.

Building a mindset for innovation is an integral part of the athletic journey that macrodosing can cultivate. In a highly competitive environment, innovation can be the key to success. Macrodosing fosters a mindset that is open to innovation and actively seeks it. This can inspire athletes to constantly evolve, experiment with new methods, and remain at the cutting edge of their sport. This mindset ensures that they are not just reacting to the game but shaping it, staying ahead of their competition through continuous innovation and growth.

In essence, macrodosing offers a gateway into a cognitive landscape where creativity, adaptability, and innovation flourish. It's a landscape that resonates with the dynamic nature of sports, where the ability to think creatively and adapt swiftly can be the difference between victory and defeat. By tapping into this potential, athletes can infuse their game with inventive techniques, fresh perspectives, and an agility that keeps them in sync with the ever-changing rhythm of competition. Fusing these elements can transform the athletic experience, elevating performance and allowing athletes to approach their sport with a vibrancy and inventiveness that sets them apart. Whether on the training ground or in the heat of competition, these enhanced cognitive abilities can be a game-changer, turning the unexpected into opportunities and the conventional into extraordinary.

Therapeutic Applications: The pressures and challenges of competitive sports can take a significant toll on athletes, often manifesting in mental health challenges such as anxiety, depression, burnout, and more. In pursuing physical excellence, the mental and emotional aspects of well-being are sometimes neglected, yet they are vital for sustained performance and overall quality of life. Macrodosing, the practice of using larger, fully psychoactive doses of psychedelics, presents a fascinating therapeutic avenue that has been gaining attention in this regard.

The profound introspective journey of a macrodosing session can serve as a therapeutic process, diving into the depths of the psyche to uncover and address underlying emotional issues. Athletes may grapple with fears of failure, pressures of performance, body image concerns, insecurities, or even deeper-rooted issues from their personal lives. Macrodosing has shown potential in guiding individuals through these emotional landscapes, offering a space to confront, understand, and begin healing these wounds. It's not merely a fleeting experience but can catalyze lasting change, reshaping an individual's emotional framework.

For athletes, the revelations and healing during a macrodosing session can translate into improved mental well-being and, consequently, better performance on the field. Facing and overcoming deep-seated fears can lead to newfound confidence and poise in competition. Healing from past traumas can lead to a more balanced and centered approach to training and competing. Addressing anxieties can lead to more focused and enjoyable engagement with the sport. The overall effect is a more resilient, centered, and joyful athlete, capable of pursuing their sport passionately and purposefully.

Professional guidance can play a critical role in harnessing the therapeutic potential of macrodosing for athletes. Therapists trained in psychedelic-assisted therapy can provide a safe and supportive environment for the macrodosing experience, guiding athletes through the process, and helping them integrate the insights and changes into their daily lives. This integration phase is vital, ensuring that the profound shifts experienced during a macrodosing session translate into actionable changes in thinking, behavior, and overall approach to life and sport.

The emotional releases during a macrodosing session are often cathartic and transformative. These are abstract experiences and have practical implications in an athlete's life. By processing emotional baggage, athletes can unburden themselves, leading to a more accessible, authentic engagement with their sport. The newfound clarity can also help them set more aligned and meaningful goals, steering their athletic journey in a direction that resonates with their true self.

The holistic well-being that macrodosing may foster extends beyond the sporting arena. The positive shifts in mental health, self-awareness, and emotional balance contribute to a higher quality of life overall. Relationships may deepen, personal growth may accelerate, and a sense of connection to oneself and the world may flourish. For an athlete, this well-rounded growth ensures that they are performing at their best and living at their best, in harmony with themselves and their surroundings.

Macrodosing presents a multifaceted therapeutic tool for athletes, capable of addressing the complex mental health challenges often accompanying the pursuit of excellence. Opening doors to profound self-insight, emotional healing, and mental balance offers a pathway to well-being that sustains not just athletic performance but the entirety of the athlete's life. It's a holistic approach that recognizes the athlete as a performer and human being, seeking balance, growth, and fulfillment. Coupled with professional guidance, macrodosing may hold a key to a new dimension of sports therapy that embraces the entire athlete's experience and paves the way for a more enlightened, compassionate, and practical approach to athletic well-being.

Community and Connection: Macrodosing's ability to forge a sense of connectedness and empathy extends into the sports domain, opening up profound opportunities for team dynamics, sportsmanship, and community building. In team sports' intense, interconnected world, the dissolution of ego boundaries often experienced during macrodosing can foster a profound connection to teammates and the surrounding environment. This connection leads to improved communication, cooperation, and synchronization on the field, transforming a group of individual athletes into a more harmonious and effective unit.

The heightened awareness of one's place within a broader context nurtures a genuine sense of sportsmanship. Competition is approached with respect, integrity, and grace, reflecting a set of ethics that values participation, mutual growth, and the joy of the game above winning or losing. The community-centric approach further weaves a supportive network that bolsters performance and overall well-being, reflecting the essence of sports as a shared journey of striving, celebrating, growing, and inspiring.

The profound connection to the natural world that often emerges from macrodosing can lead to more sustainable practices within training and lifestyle. It enhances the sensory and spiritual connection to the physical spaces where sports are played, adding deeper meaning to the athletic pursuit.

By nurturing empathy, connection, sportsmanship, and environmental stewardship, macrodosing supports the evolution of a sports culture rooted in mutual respect, shared purpose, joy, and holistic well-being. This vision of sports intertwines competition and excellence with compassion, integrity, and personal growth, presenting a holistic, human-centered approach where the pursuit of excellence is connected to the values of respect and shared humanity.

Together, these aspects contribute to a transformative path toward a more compassionate and meaningful embodiment of sports. By integrating macrodosing into a responsible and guided approach to athletic development, athletes can tap into a more profound, more connected way of engaging with their sport, teammates, and themselves.

The power of macrodosing reaches far beyond a fleeting psychedelic experience. It offers a pathway to profound, lasting personal growth and self-understanding, with wide-ranging implications for athletes. From dismantling mental barriers and strengthening resilience to aligning personal values and enhancing creativity, macrodosing can be a profound tool in an athlete's toolkit. It invites athletes to explore the depths of their psyche, unlock hidden potentials, and embark on a fulfilling and enlightened athletic journey. As the dialogue around psychedelics continues to evolve, exploring macrodosing to enhance not just athletic performance but the entirety of the human experience remains a thrilling frontier.

Overcoming Mental Blocks and Fears

The journey towards peak athletic performance is as much a mental endeavor as it is physical. One of the prominent barriers that athletes often confront is the entanglement of mental blocks, fears, lack of confidence, anxiety, and stress. These psychological impediments can stem from deeply ingrained beliefs, past failures, self-imposed limitations, or societal pressure to perform. They can manifest in various ways, hindering an athlete's progress and stifling their true potential.

Macrodosing magic mushrooms introduces an innovative and potentially transformative avenue to address these mental challenges directly. The experience induced is unlike any traditional therapeutic approach. It plunges the athlete into heightened awareness, altered perception, and profound introspection. This unique mental landscape provides an opportunity to view personal challenges from a fresh perspective, breaking free from conventional thought patterns and enabling the recognition and dismantling of mental obstacles.

During a guided macrodosing session, the emergence of vivid imagery, raw emotions, or suppressed memories may lead to astonishing insights into the root causes of anxieties and fears. These revelations allow athletes to face and understand the very core of what has been holding them back. Encountering these fears in a controlled, supportive, and therapeutically guided environment, athletes can work through them, process their underlying emotions, and reduce or even eradicate their negative impact on performance.

However, the benefits of macrodosing extend beyond mere confrontation and resolution. The experience often fosters interconnectedness, unity, and empathy with others and oneself. This deeper self-connection encourages the development of self-compassion, a powerful ally in overcoming fears, self-doubt, and performance anxiety. Embracing self-compassion is not about denying weaknesses or failures; instead, it's about acknowledging them as part of the human experience and responding to oneself with understanding and kindness.

This compassionate relationship with oneself is instrumental in cultivating resilience, boosting self-esteem, and instilling a renewed sense of confidence. Athletes may find themselves empowered to approach their sport with a mindset untethered by prior limitations, driven by intrinsic motivation, and resilient in the face of adversity.

Furthermore, the profound realizations gained through macrodosing can have far-reaching effects on an athlete's overall life philosophy, aligning their sporting pursuits with broader life goals and values. This alignment brings meaning and purpose to their athletic journey, transforming it into a fulfilling path of self-discovery and growth.

In summary, macrodosing offers a multifaceted approach to mental optimization that goes beyond traditional sports psychology. By unlocking the inner chambers of the mind, it provides an extraordinary tool for self-exploration, mental liberation, and personal empowerment. It has the potential to reshape an athlete's mental framework, turning previously insurmountable barriers into surmountable challenges, and imbuing the athletic journey with richness, depth, and a profound sense of humanity. It's a pathway that demands respect, understanding, and professional guidance but opens up uncharted territories for those willing to explore.

Enhancing Mind-body Connection

The realm of sports is an exquisite dance between the mind and the body. Every stride, stroke, or swing is a harmonious blend of physical execution and mental direction. Enhancing this mind-body connection is paramount for athletes aiming for optimal performance, and macrodosing magic mushrooms emerges as an intriguing method to cultivate this vital connection.

A strong mind-body connection manifests in a heightened awareness of one's physical sensations, movements, and overall bodily state. This awareness enables athletes to respond precisely to the physical demands of their training and competition. Macrodosing psilocybin can induce an altered state of consciousness that sharpens this connection, providing insights that transcend the usual sensory perception.

During a guided macrodosing session, individuals may become exquisitely sensitive to nuances such as muscle tension, breath rhythm, heart rate, and even the subtle energy flow within the body. This sensitivity is not just an abstract experience but can be translated into tangible benefits in the athletic context.

Firstly, a heightened awareness can lead to better body control and understanding. Athletes may develop an improved sense of biomechanics, understanding how each muscle, joint, and ligament interacts in a complex symphony of movement. This newfound comprehension can facilitate movement efficiency, coordination, and grace, whether executing a perfect golf swing, a gymnastic routine, or an explosive sprint.

Secondly, the ability to intuitively gauge one's physical limits can lead to more effective and safe training. Athletes can learn to push their boundaries without crossing into the danger zone that risks injury or burnout. This sense of bodily intuition is akin to an internal compass, guiding athletes through the challenging landscape of intense physical training.

Furthermore, the enhanced mind-body connection fosters a profound sense of presence and focus. This presence transcends mere concentration; it's a state of being wholly engaged in the present moment, where distractions fade away, and a calm determination takes over. This mental state is invaluable during high-stakes competitions, where pressure, excitement, and external expectations can quickly derail focus. Athletes with a robust mind-body connection can remain anchored in the moment, managing distractions, maintaining composure, and executing their strategies with fluidity and poise.

Incorporating macrodosing sessions into an athlete's training regimen is more than just an experimental approach; it's an organized and thoughtful integration of a powerful tool that can unlock dimensions of human potential often untouched by traditional training methods. It requires guidance, preparation, and an understanding of the profound nature of the psychedelic experience.

In conclusion, enhancing the mind-body connection through macrodosing opens up a realm of possibilities for athletes. It's a holistic approach that nurtures the physical prowess and the mental and emotional aspects inseparable from peak performance. Whether it's the subtle grace of a dancer, the explosive power of a sprinter, or the strategic mind of a chess player, the enhanced connection between mind and body can be a transformative element in the pursuit of excellence, and macrodosing offers a unique pathway to explore and cultivate this connection.

Creating a Supportive Set and Setting for Macrodosing Sessions

Creating a supportive set and setting for macrodosing sessions is crucial for athletes seeking to harness the full potential of magic mushrooms for personal growth and performance enhancement. Set and setting refer to the mindset (set) and the environment (setting) in which an individual experiences a psychedelic substance. Both factors can significantly influence the nature and outcome of the experience.

Set refers to the mental and emotional state of the individual before the macrodosing session. It includes their beliefs, expectations, and intentions regarding the experience. To ensure a positive and productive session, athletes must approach the experience with a clear intention, an open mind, and a positive attitude. Some helpful strategies to prepare for a macrodosing session include setting specific goals for personal growth, practicing relaxation techniques, and engaging in activities that promote a positive mindset.

On the other hand, setting refers to the physical and social environment in which the macrodosing session occurs. Creating a comfortable, safe, and supportive space that allows the individual to engage with the experience without distraction or anxiety is vital. Considerations for an optimal setting include:

1. Choosing a familiar and comfortable location, such as a private room or a quiet outdoor space.
2. Ensuring the space is clean, organized, and free of potential hazards or distractions.
3. Providing access to comforting items, such as blankets, pillows, or soothing music.
4. Ensuring privacy and limiting interruptions from others.
5. Having a trusted friend, family member, or therapist present to provide support and guidance if needed.

By carefully considering and preparing the set and setting, athletes can increase the likelihood of having a positive and transformative macrodosing experience, ultimately contributing to their growth and performance enhancement.

Personal Experiences and Case Studies

This section will explore personal experiences and case studies of athletes who have utilized macrodosing magic mushrooms to achieve transformative breakthroughs in their performance and personal growth. These real-life examples demonstrate the potential benefits and challenges of macrodosing for athletic purposes.

A professional cyclist, Sarah struggled with anxiety and self-doubt that hindered her performance in high-pressure races. After a series of macrodosing sessions, she experienced a shift in her mindset, allowing her to overcome her fears and develop a newfound confidence in her abilities. As a result, Sarah broke through her mental barriers and achieved personal bests in her races.

Mark, a weightlifter, turned to macrodosing to address a plateau in his training progress. During his sessions, he could identify and confront deep-seated beliefs about his limitations and self-worth holding him back. By working through these issues, Mark was able to unlock new levels of strength and resilience, leading to significant gains in his lifting performance.

A marathon runner, Emily faced ongoing issues with injury and chronic pain. Through macrodosing sessions, she developed a greater awareness of the mind-body connection, allowing her to understand better and manage her pain. This newfound perspective and a more holistic approach to training and recovery led to improved injury prevention and a faster return to running after setbacks.

A professional swimmer, Laura struggled with burnout and a lack of motivation after years of intense training. Hoping to reignite her passion for the sport, she decided to try macrodosing magic mushrooms. During her sessions, Laura connected with her love for swimming and rediscovered the joy she once found in competition. As a result, she was able to rekindle her enthusiasm and improve her performance in the pool.

Daniel, a basketball player, had been experiencing difficulties maintaining team cohesion and communication on the court. After several macrodosing sessions, Daniel found that his empathy and emotional intelligence were significantly enhanced. This allowed him to understand his teammates' perspectives better and foster a more supportive team dynamic, leading to improved on-court chemistry and overall team performance.

Samantha, a gymnast, faced challenges in managing the stress and expectations that came with her sport. She turned to macrodosing magic mushrooms in hopes of finding a way to cope with the pressure. Through her sessions, Samantha developed mindfulness techniques and a deeper understanding of her emotional triggers, allowing her to manage her stress more effectively. This ultimately led to greater consistency in her performances and a more fulfilling gymnastics experience.

A professional golfer, James struggled with performance anxiety that negatively impacted his game. By incorporating macrodosing into his routine, James was able to address the root causes of his anxiety and develop mental strategies to remain calm and focused under pressure. This newfound mental resilience significantly improved his golf game, leading to better tournament results and greater overall satisfaction with his performance.

Maria, a competitive cyclist, faced a plateau in her performance, struggling to reach new personal records despite rigorous training. After trying macrodosing with magic mushrooms, Maria gained insights into the mental barriers holding her back. She overcame these obstacles by overcoming her performance plateau and setting new personal records.

Kevin, an endurance runner, had been coping with a fear of failure, affecting his ability to reach his full potential. Through macrodosing sessions, Kevin confronted and addressed the root of his fear. This newfound mental clarity allowed him to approach his races, leading to improved race times confidently and a more enjoyable running experience.

Emily, a professional dancer, had been dealing with a lack of creativity and struggled to find inspiration for her choreography. After incorporating macrodosing with magic mushrooms into her routine, Emily experienced a surge of creative energy and renewed passion for her art. This ultimately led to more innovative and captivating dance performances.

These case studies illustrate how macrodosing magic mushrooms can support athletes in overcoming mental blocks, enhancing the mind-body connection, and achieving transformative breakthroughs in their performance. While individual experiences will vary, these examples provide valuable insights into the potential benefits of incorporating macrodosing into an athlete's training regimen.

Combining Magic Mushrooms with Other Performance Enhancers

In the dynamic and fiercely competitive world of sports, athletes continually seek innovative ways to push the boundaries of their abilities. Utilizing performance-enhancing substances is not new; however, incorporating magic mushrooms into this sphere represents an intriguing frontier in athletic performance optimization. In this chapter, we will delve into the complex interplay between magic mushrooms and other performance enhancers, shedding light on the synergistic effects that may lead to significant improvements in both physical and mental prowess.

Synergy refers to the cooperative interaction between different substances, leading to an effect more significant than the sum of their contributions. When applied to athletic performance, the synergy concept explores how combining magic mushrooms with various legal and illegal performance enhancers can amplify the effects, often unlocking benefits that may be unattainable with the substances used independently.

We will explore these synergistic effects comprehensively, scrutinizing different combinations, such as magic mushrooms with stimulants like caffeine, cognitive enhancers like nootropics, adaptogens for stress management, and even traditional performance enhancers like creatine. The chapter will delve into the mechanics of how these combinations might work, offering insights into these synergies' biological, psychological, and physiological dimensions.

Safety, of course, is paramount. While the prospect of amplified benefits is tempting, it also comes with potential risks. Careful experimentation, meticulous monitoring, and a comprehensive understanding of possible side effects are essential to navigating this complex terrain. The chapter will guide the responsible exploration of these combinations, emphasizing the importance of individualized approaches and professional oversight.

Moreover, we will venture into the equally crucial arena of nutrition and supplements. The role of a balanced diet, key nutrients, hydration, and electrolytes are all fundamental components in the athletic performance equation. Understanding how magic mushrooms may interact with these aspects, possibly impacting nutrient absorption and utilization, adds another layer of complexity to this fascinating subject.

Finally, the chapter will stress the importance of a personalized approach. Every athlete has unique needs, goals, genetic factors, and responses to different substances. We will discuss how athletes can assess and monitor their personal experiences, continually fine-tuning their strategies to find the optimal combination of enhancers. This approach requires collaboration with professionals and experts in sports performance and nutrition, as the intersection between magic mushrooms and other enhancers is an intricate field, demanding a nuanced understanding.

In conclusion, Chapter 4 represents a pioneering exploration into the synergistic world of magic mushrooms and other performance enhancers. It is a complex and multifaceted journey that opens up new horizons for athletes seeking to transcend their limitations. By thoughtfully combining different substances and aligning them with individual goals and values, athletes can approach their pursuit of excellence with creativity, wisdom, and integrity. The ethical considerations, potential risks, and personal variability make this an area filled with opportunity and responsibility, and this chapter aims to be a comprehensive guide for those daring to venture into this exciting frontier of human potential.

The Synergistic Effect of Combining Substances

In the intricate landscape of performance enhancement, synergy is a concept that offers a unique and potentially powerful pathway to optimize athletic abilities. Synergy refers to the phenomenon where the combined effect of two or more substances is greater than the sum of their individual effects. This interplay can result in amplified benefits, allowing athletes to reach new heights in their performance.

Combining magic mushrooms with other performance enhancers is a cutting-edge approach that may hold untapped potential. Through careful integration and understanding of how different substances interact, athletes can explore innovative strategies to push their boundaries. This section delves into the concept of synergy in performance enhancement, exploring how magic mushrooms can amplify the effects of other performance enhancers, and highlighting the importance of careful experimentation and monitoring for potential side effects.

The pursuit of synergy is a complex task. It demands a profound understanding of the substances involved, a meticulous approach to dosing and timing, and a keen awareness of the individual's physiological response. By demystifying the synergistic effect of combining magic mushrooms with other enhancers, athletes, and professionals can open new doors to performance optimization while navigating the associated complexities and responsibilities.

Understanding the concept of synergy in performance enhancement

The concept of synergy refers to the collaborative interaction between two or more substances, creating a combined effect that surpasses the individual impact of each substance on its own. In the realm of athletic performance enhancement, the application of synergy has taken on a pivotal role, offering a new frontier of possibilities for athletes striving to reach their peak potential. When substances are utilized synergistically, they can produce unique and amplified benefits that would otherwise be unattainable when used separately.

Synergy's foundation lies in the understanding that substances can have complementary actions, amplifying each other's effectiveness. For example, one substance might enhance energy levels while another improves focus. Together, they could provide a heightened mental and physical readiness beyond what either could achieve alone. This harmonious interaction opens up opportunities for more precise tailoring of performance-enhancement strategies, enabling athletes to target specific aspects of their physical and mental capabilities with unprecedented precision.

Yet, the world of synergistic effects is complex and nuanced, demanding a thorough understanding of the individual substances involved, their mechanisms of action, and how they interact. The science behind these interactions is still unfolding, and the subject is ripe for exploration and study. Ongoing research is crucial to uncover the full spectrum of possibilities synergy offers, guiding athletes and professionals in their pursuit of excellence. Athletes must approach synergy with caution and awareness, recognizing that while the rewards may be great, the path is intricate and must be navigated with care and expertise. Through careful study, consultation with professionals, and personalized experimentation, the potential of synergy in performance enhancement can be unlocked, heralding a new era of athletic achievement.

How magic mushrooms can amplify the effects of other performance enhancers

Magic mushrooms, specifically those containing the psychoactive compound psilocybin, have increasingly been recognized for their potential to enhance human performance. When combined with other performance enhancers, the synergy achieved can be pretty remarkable, potentially leading to amplified effects catering to athletic endeavors' specific demands.

The synergistic interaction between magic mushrooms and other performance-enhancing substances arises from the distinct ways they can influence the mind and body. For example, magic mushrooms promote introspection, creativity, and mental clarity, while other enhancers might boost physical energy, endurance, or cognitive speed. When used together, these substances can create a multifaceted approach to performance optimization, allowing athletes to target various aspects of their training and competition simultaneously.

The profound psychological effects of magic mushrooms can further enhance the effects of other substances by fostering a greater connection to one's physical state, enabling more accurate tuning to the body's needs, whether enhancing the focus provided by stimulants or deepening the relaxation and recovery promoted by adaptogens, magic mushrooms in a synergistic combination can enrich the overall experience.

The ability of magic mushrooms to induce altered states of consciousness may provide athletes with novel perspectives on their training, opening up new avenues for growth and breaking through insurmountable mental barriers. These enhanced insights can guide more efficient and targeted use of other performance enhancers, resulting in a more cohesive and comprehensive approach to improvement.

However, combining magic mushrooms with other performance enhancers has its complexities. Understanding the pharmacology, dosage, timing, and potential interactions between substances is crucial to avoid unexpected side effects or diminished benefits. Personalized guidance and carefully controlled experimentation under professional supervision are essential to navigate this uncharted territory. Combining magic mushrooms with other performance enhancers is a burgeoning field of exploration, offering a compelling yet intricate landscape that promises to redefine the boundaries of athletic potential.

The importance of careful experimentation and monitoring for potential side effects

The world of synergistic performance enhancement, especially involving magic mushrooms and other potent substances, is filled with exciting opportunities and significant risks. The interplay between different compounds can lead to effects that are not only amplified but also unpredictable. As such, careful experimentation and monitoring for potential side effects are paramount to maintaining safety and effectiveness.

Magic mushrooms have a complex profile of psychological effects, and when combined with other performance enhancers, the potential interactions can become multifaceted and hard to predict. Different substances may interact to enhance or negate each other's effects, and individual responses can vary widely. This complexity necessitates a cautious approach, involving gradual experimentation, meticulous documentation of experiences, and keen observation for unexpected physiological or psychological responses.

Professional guidance is often indispensable in this process, as experts in the fields of sports medicine, nutrition, and even psychedelics can provide valuable insights into safe practices, appropriate dosages, and potential contraindications. Collaboration with professionals ensures experimentation is grounded in scientific understanding and aligned with individual goals and physiological characteristics.

Monitoring for side effects must be an ongoing process. Athletes should be aware of short-term and long-term effects, including possible impacts on mental health, physical performance, recovery, and overall well-being. Regular assessments and reflection on personal experiences are vital in recognizing any emerging patterns or concerns.

The exploration of synergistic effects between magic mushrooms and other performance enhancers is a journey that offers incredible potential for athletic growth but requires a conscientious and informed approach. Careful experimentation and continuous monitoring are essential to unlocking the benefits while minimizing the risks, reflecting a responsible and enlightened pursuit of excellence. The role of professionals, adherence to legal guidelines, and a strong focus on individual well-being must guide this adventurous path to new frontiers in sports performance.

Safe and Effective Combinations for Athletes

Athletic excellence is not merely about pushing the body to its limits but doing so in a safe, sustainable way, and in line with the athlete's unique needs and goals. Integrating magic mushrooms with other performance enhancers can offer a multifaceted approach to achieving peak performance. Still, it requires an understanding of the specific combinations that are both effective and safe.

This section explores the various substances and strategies that can be combined with magic mushrooms, each with its own potential benefits and considerations. From traditional performance enhancers like creatine to modern nootropics and even common stimulants like caffeine, there are diverse options available for athletes to explore.

However, these combinations are not one-size-fits-all. What works wonders for one athlete may be ineffective or even harmful for another. Therefore, it becomes crucial to understand the nuances of these combinations, their impact on the body, and how they align with an athlete's unique physiology and goals.

Whether boosting energy and focus, enhancing cognitive function, or aiding in stress management and recovery, the combinations discussed in this section are designed to guide athletes toward an individualized and holistic approach to performance enhancement. By exploring the safe and effective synergies between magic mushrooms and other substances, athletes can create tailored strategies that elevate their performance while prioritizing their well-being.

Combining magic mushrooms with caffeine or other stimulants for increased energy and focus

The integration of magic mushrooms with caffeine or other stimulants presents an intriguing area of exploration for athletes seeking to enhance their energy and focus. While each substance has distinct effects, the combination may synergistically amplify these attributes to provide a unique boost in performance.

Magic mushrooms, particularly in macrodosing, can induce heightened awareness and introspection, while caffeine and other stimulants are known for increasing alertness and energy levels. When combined, these substances might create a balanced and enhanced mental state, where magic mushrooms' profound insights and self-awareness meld with the invigoration and concentration provided by stimulants.

This combination is challenging. The potent effects of stimulants like caffeine might conflict with or overshadow the more subtle and nuanced effects of magic mushrooms. This potential clash requires a careful balance and precise dosing to harness the desired synergistic effects without causing discomfort or negating the benefits of either substance.

Athletes who wish to experiment with this combination should do so with caution, starting with lower doses and paying close attention to the timing of consumption. It might be beneficial to combine these substances during specific training sessions where heightened focus and increased energy are required, rather than during recovery or more contemplative periods.

Professional guidance can also be invaluable in this process, as experts in sports nutrition and performance enhancement can help tailor the combination to an individual's specific needs, performance goals, and physiological response. Additionally, monitoring for potential side effects, such as increased heart rate, anxiety, or digestive issues, is vital to ensure safety and effectiveness.

Ethical and legal considerations must always be considered, particularly concerning stimulants that might be prohibited or restricted in competitive sports. Athletes should thoroughly research and adhere to their specific sport's rules and regulations to avoid potential disqualifications or legal issues.

Combining magic mushrooms with caffeine or other stimulants represents a promising avenue for athletes seeking to enhance their energy and focus. Yet, this complex synergy requires a thoughtful and responsible approach, balancing the unique attributes of each substance, considering individual needs, and complying with legal and ethical standards. With proper guidance, experimentation, and vigilance, athletes may unlock new levels of performance through this novel and stimulating combination.

Using magic mushrooms alongside nootropics to enhance cognitive function

Combining magic mushrooms with nootropics represents an exciting frontier in cognitive enhancement for athletes. Nootropics, often called "smart drugs," include various substances designed to boost cognitive function, improve memory, and creativity, and increase focus. When used alongside magic mushrooms, the synergistic effects can be profound.

Magic mushrooms, primarily through their active compound psilocybin, have been linked to heightened creativity and a more fluid thought process. Combining them with specific nootropics that target focus and cognitive clarity can create a balanced and potent mix. For instance, modafinil may sharpen concentration, while the Racetam family of nootropics can improve memory and learning capacity.

This synergy between magic mushrooms and nootropics can enhance mental acuity and decision-making skills for athletes. It can provide a heightened awareness of the game's dynamics, more rapid adaptation to unexpected scenarios, and a more profound strategic insight. This combination could be a game-changer in sports where split-second decisions can make the difference between victory and defeat.

However, combining these substances has its challenges and risks. Navigating the complex world of nootropics requires a clear understanding of each substance's properties, potential interactions, and appropriate dosing. Athletes must also know the legal status of various nootropics within their jurisdiction and respective sports governing bodies.

Consulting with professionals experienced in sports nutrition or neuropharmacology is advisable to create a personalized plan that aligns with an athlete's specific needs and complies with all relevant regulations. In addition, ongoing monitoring and adjustments may be required to fine-tune the combination and ensure it supports the athlete's goals without adverse effects.

Ultimately, blending magic mushrooms with nootropics offers a fascinating avenue for cognitive enhancement in sports, opening doors to new levels of mental prowess and strategic mastery. However, this path requires careful navigation, informed decisions, and a willingness to engage with these substances' complexity and interactions.

Examples of Nootropics for Synergistic Use with Magic Mushrooms

Racetams (Piracetam, Aniracetam, etc.): Racetams are a well-known family of nootropics for improving memory, learning, and cognition. When paired with magic mushrooms, they may amplify creative thinking and problem-solving skills, providing athletes with enhanced mental agility.

Modafinil: A popular stimulant used for wakefulness, Modafinil has been found to increase focus and cognitive function. Combining it with magic mushrooms may increase energy levels and sustained concentration, which is instrumental in endurance sports or training sessions.

L-Theanine: Often found in tea, L-Theanine is known for promoting relaxation without drowsiness. When used with magic mushrooms, it might balance the psychedelic experience, providing calmness and clarity, enhancing mindfulness, and aiding in stress management during competitions.

Alpha-GPC (Choline source): Alpha-GPC is a precursor to acetylcholine, a memory and muscle control neurotransmitter. Its combination with magic mushrooms could enhance the mind-body connection and improve mental and physical coordination.

Bacopa Monnieri: This herb is traditionally used for enhancing memory and cognitive function. Together with magic mushrooms, it may synergistically affect cognitive flexibility, adaptability, and resilience under pressure.

Rhodiola Rosea: Known for its adaptogenic properties, Rhodiola can help with stress resistance and fatigue. When paired with magic mushrooms, the combination might promote mental and physical endurance, support recovery, and optimize overall performance.

Noopept: This synthetic compound promotes neural communication and cognitive function. It might be used with magic mushrooms to enhance further mental clarity, memory recall, and creative insight.

Ginkgo Biloba: Renowned for its ability to increase blood flow to the brain, Ginkgo Biloba may amplify the cognitive-enhancing effects of magic mushrooms, boosting concentration and information processing speed.

Lion's Mane Mushroom: Interestingly, this edible mushroom has nootropic properties and is known to support nerve growth factors. Combining it with magic mushrooms might boost neural plasticity, facilitating learning and adaptation to new strategies and techniques in sports.

Ashwagandha: As another adaptogen, Ashwagandha may reduce stress and anxiety. Paired with magic mushrooms, it could help athletes manage the psychological pressures of competition, fostering mental stability and resilience.

Oxiracetam: Known to enhance memory and learning abilities, Oxiracetam may complement the reflective aspects of magic mushrooms, promoting cognitive clarity.

Centrophenoxine: This nootropic has been used to combat cognitive decline and may synergize with magic mushrooms to promote mental alertness and memory retention.

PRL-8-53: As a powerful memory enhancer, PRL-8-53 might be paired with magic mushrooms to support long-term memory formation and cognitive processing.

Sunifiram: This novel ampakine nootropic may work well with magic mushrooms to heighten focus, decision-making abilities, and mental energy.

Coluracetam: Recognized for its potential to boost mood and creativity, Coluracetam might complement the reflective qualities of a magic mushroom experience.

Fasoracetam: As a nootropic that may aid in focus and relaxation, Fasoracetam could work synergistically with magic mushrooms to deepen the meditative aspects of the experience.

Uridine Monophosphate: Known to support overall brain health and synaptic function, Uridine may pair well with magic mushrooms to enhance neural connectivity and cognitive function.

Picamilon: This combination of GABA and niacin might be used with magic mushrooms to promote relaxation and mental clarity, enhancing the emotional aspects of the experience.

Idebenone: A synthetic analog of CoQ10, Idebenone might be paired with magic mushrooms to support cellular energy production and cognitive vitality.

Bacopa Monnieri: Though often considered an adaptogen, Bacopa Monnieri has notable nootropic effects and might synergize with magic mushrooms to enhance memory and reduce anxiety.

While the above examples provide promising avenues for exploration, it's essential to stress that combining these substances should be approached with caution and ideally under the guidance of a knowledgeable healthcare provider. The synergistic effects can vary significantly between individuals, and the appropriate selection and dosing require careful consideration of an athlete's unique needs, goals, and the rules of their respective sports governing bodies.

Incorporating adaptogens stress management and recovery

Incorporating adaptogens with magic mushrooms offers a nuanced approach to stress management and recovery for athletes. Adaptogens are special herbs or botanical compounds that help the body adapt to physical, emotional, and mental stress. Their unique qualities make them attractive to athletes who often grapple with the pressures of intense training, competition, and the constant need for peak performance.

The synergy between adaptogens and the reflective qualities of a macrodosing session with magic mushrooms could create a holistic sense of well-being. Adaptogens may support calming effects on the nervous system, reduce cortisol levels, and enhance mood, which can be invaluable for athletes. When coupled with magic mushrooms, these effects may deepen, promoting a sense of balance, mental clarity, and a more profound connection to one's physical and emotional state. This tandem can lead to enhanced self-awareness, enabling athletes to better understand their physical limitations and recovery needs.

The combination of adaptogens and magic mushrooms may also aid in improving endurance, mental focus, and recuperation from physical strain. The adaptogenic properties could assist in reducing inflammation, boosting immune function, and optimizing overall recovery, while the psychedelic experience may foster a more intuitive and practical approach to training and self-care.

This innovative pathway, targeting both mental and physical aspects of performance, offers a comprehensive approach to stress management, recovery, and self-awareness. As this is a highly individualized and nuanced area, athletes considering this approach should seek proper guidance and be mindful of their specific needs and the potential legal and ethical considerations within their sport. Exploring the integration of adaptogens with magic mushrooms could enhance performance, greater resilience, and a more profound, more meaningful athletic journey.

Examples of Adaptogens for Synergistic Use with Magic Mushrooms

Ashwagandha: This adaptogen is known for its anxiety-reducing effects, which may align with the calming aspects of magic mushrooms. By potentially reducing cortisol levels, ashwagandha could contribute to a more profound and reflective experience, aiding athletes in addressing stress and recovery needs.

Rhodiola Rosea: Often used to boost physical endurance and combat mental fatigue, Rhodiola may complement the mind-body connection fostered during a magic mushroom experience. For athletes, this combination could enhance focus, energy, and resilience.

Ginseng: With its well-researched effects on energy levels and cognitive function, ginseng could be a valuable addition to the macrodosing experience. It may help athletes tap into greater concentration and mental clarity, potentially magnifying the creative and adaptive thinking associated with psilocybin.

Cordyceps: These medicinal mushrooms have been reported to improve stamina and support adrenal function. Alongside magic mushrooms, cordyceps offer athletes a pathway to increased energy and recovery support.

Holy Basil (Tulsi): Known for its calming and anti-inflammatory properties, it could pair well with magic mushrooms to nurture a relaxed, receptive state, supporting emotional release and mental clarity.

Schisandra: This berry has been used to reduce stress and improve performance under pressure. It could synergize with magic mushrooms to further boost an athlete's mental resilience and focus.

Reishi Mushroom: Although not an adaptogen in the traditional sense, Reishi shares similar balancing effects and might complement magic mushrooms to deepen relaxation and enhance immune function.

Astragalus: Known for its immune-boosting and anti-inflammatory properties, Astragalus might be a suitable partner with magic mushrooms, enhancing overall well-being and potentially aiding recovery.

Maca Root: Often hailed for its energy-boosting and hormone-balancing effects, Maca could work harmoniously with magic mushrooms to amplify physical endurance and support a balanced emotional state.

Siberian Ginseng (Eleuthero): This adaptogen, known for increasing stamina and fighting fatigue, could align with the mind-body connection fostered by magic mushrooms, possibly leading to greater resilience and focus in athletes.

Licorice Root: Recognized for its soothing effect on the digestive and respiratory systems, Licorice Root could complement the introspective and calming effects of magic mushrooms, helping athletes manage stress and promote overall wellness.

Gotu Kola: This herb, traditionally used to enhance memory and nervous system function, might synergize with magic mushrooms to foster deeper introspection, creativity, and cognitive clarity.

Moringa: Known for its rich nutrient content, Moringa might provide a nutritional complement to magic mushrooms, supporting overall health, energy levels, and recovery.

Suma Root: Also known as "Brazilian ginseng," Suma Root may help with fatigue and stress, possibly aligning well with magic mushrooms to enhance mental and physical performance.

Bacopa Monnieri: Often used to enhance cognitive function and alleviate anxiety, Bacopa could synergize with magic mushrooms to deepen introspection and support mental clarity and calmness.

Ginkgo Biloba: With its potential to improve circulation and cognitive function, Ginkgo might be a suitable partner with magic mushrooms, aiding focus, memory, and overall mental acuity.

The Role of Nutrition and Supplements in Optimizing Performance

In athletics, the emphasis often falls on training regimens, physical skills, and psychological conditioning. However, nutrition and supplementation are equally vital in supporting and enhancing athletic performance. While magic mushrooms offer a range of benefits that may augment mental and emotional aspects, understanding how they interact with the body's nutritional needs and how they might be combined with dietary strategies is key to realizing their full potential. In this section, we will explore the fundamental principles of nutrition and supplementation for athletes, examining how a balanced diet, essential nutrients, hydration, and magic mushrooms can all synergize to create an optimal environment for performance. From energy production and muscle growth to maintaining peak performance during intense training or competition, these factors work together in a complex interplay that demands careful consideration and tailored approaches. Whether you are a professional athlete or a fitness enthusiast, the insights in this section will offer valuable guidance on how to nourish and fuel your body in harmony with your goals and the unique attributes of magic mushrooms.

The importance of a balanced diet for athletic performance

A balanced diet is the cornerstone of any athlete's performance and recovery, providing the essential nutrients required to fuel the body, repair tissues, and maintain optimal health. While training regimens and performance enhancers like magic mushrooms can offer targeted benefits, the nourishment derived from a balanced diet lays the foundation for success.

In athletics, a balanced diet is not merely about consuming a variety of foods; it's about precisely calibrating the intake of proteins, carbohydrates, fats, vitamins, and minerals to meet the unique demands of the athlete's sport and individual physiology. Proteins support muscle growth and repair, carbohydrates provide quick energy, fats ensure long-term energy reserves, and micronutrients regulate countless biochemical processes that sustain performance.

The interplay between diet and magic mushrooms may introduce additional complexities. As substances that can deeply affect consciousness and perception, magic mushrooms may alter an athlete's relationship with food or sensitivity to nutritional needs. Understanding these potential interactions is crucial for anyone considering incorporating magic mushrooms into their performance strategy.

Furthermore, magic mushrooms may amplify the mental focus and clarity needed to adhere to a carefully designed dietary plan. This heightened awareness might allow athletes to tune into their bodies more acutely, recognizing subtle cues related to hunger, fullness, and nutritional imbalances.

For athletes seeking to explore the synergistic potential between magic mushrooms and dietary practices, collaboration with nutrition experts, who are familiar with traditional sports nutrition and the unique attributes of psychedelics, may be invaluable. By crafting a personalized diet that considers the athlete's sport, training cycle, body composition, and any psychedelic interventions, they can help ensure that all nutritional bases are covered.

A balanced diet is essential for athletic performance, providing the energy, nutrients, and support required for peak physical and mental functioning. When considered alongside the potential benefits and challenges of magic mushrooms, it's clear that nutrition is not a static or isolated aspect of athletic preparation but an integral, dynamic part of a complex performance ecosystem. By recognizing and respecting this interconnectedness, athletes can nourish themselves in a way that supports their goals and complements their use of magic mushrooms, leading to a more holistic and practical approach to performance enhancement.

Essential nutrients and supplements to support energy production and muscle growth

Energy production and muscle growth are fundamental to athletic performance, and achieving optimal levels of both requires targeted nutritional strategies. While a well-balanced diet provides the base for supporting these physiological processes, the inclusion of specific nutrients and supplements can further refine and enhance an athlete's capabilities.

Carbohydrates: As the primary fuel source for many types of exercise, carbohydrates are essential for providing immediate energy. Consuming complex carbohydrates like whole grains and legumes offers a sustained energy release, powering endurance, and intensive training sessions.

Proteins: Protein supports muscle growth and repair, vital for athletes engaged in strength training and those needing to recover from rigorous physical activities. High-quality protein sources, such as lean meats, fish, eggs, and plant-based alternatives, can help fulfill these needs.

Fats: Essential fatty acids, including omega-3 and omega-6, play a critical role in long-term energy storage and cellular function. Incorporating healthy fats from sources like avocados, nuts, and fatty fish can support overall energy metabolism.

Creatine: This supplement is well-known for its ability to enhance strength, increase lean muscle mass, and help muscles recover more quickly during exercise. Its use in combination with magic mushrooms requires careful consideration, as interactions and synergistic effects might be possible.

Amino Acids: Branched-chain amino acids (BCAAs) and other essential amino acids can further support muscle growth and recovery. Supplements containing these can be precious for athletes with high protein requirements.

Vitamins and Minerals: Micronutrients like B vitamins, Vitamin D, iron, magnesium, and zinc are essential in various metabolic processes that enable energy production and muscle function. Individual supplementation might be needed depending on the athlete's diet and sport.

Electrolytes: Sodium, potassium, and magnesium are vital in muscle contraction and energy utilization. Specialized electrolyte supplements may be necessary for athletes with prolonged or intense physical exertion.

Hydration: Though not a nutrient per se, proper hydration is paramount for energy production and muscle function. Water supports every metabolic process and must be consumed appropriately, especially during heavy training or competition.

Magic Mushrooms' Interaction with Nutrients: Magic mushrooms' interaction with nutrients is a complex aspect that requires consideration, particularly when integrated into an athletic context. The psychedelic compound psilocybin, found in magic mushrooms, has been known to affect the gastrointestinal system, leading to feelings of nausea or other digestive discomfort for some individuals. This reaction could influence the absorption of essential nutrients such as carbohydrates, proteins, fats, vitamins, and minerals, altering how the body assimilates and utilizes them. It is essential to recognize how these interactions may affect athletic performance and make the necessary dietary adjustments to mitigate any negative impacts.

Furthermore, the possible impact on gut microbiota could have long-term implications on digestion and nutrient utilization, which are still not fully understood. Research into how magic mushrooms interact with the gut's microbial environment could provide insight into optimizing diet and supplementation strategies when using these psychedelics. Understanding the underlying mechanisms can lead to more targeted nutritional approaches that complement the effects of magic mushrooms.

The psychedelic experience also induces changes in appetite, either suppressing or enhancing hunger. These shifts in eating patterns can impact energy levels and muscle growth by modifying the intake of essential nutrients required for these biological processes. Athletes considering magic mushrooms as a part of their regimen must be conscious of these fluctuations and prepare for potential changes in their eating habits and nutritional needs.

Finally, even hydration and electrolytes could be affected, given the heightened bodily sensations often reported during a psychedelic experience. The athlete may become more acutely aware of thirst or hydration levels, leading to alterations in drinking habits. This awareness may positively guide hydration strategies during training and competition but requires careful management to prevent over or under-hydration.

The dynamic relationship between magic mushrooms and nutrient absorption and utilization opens a fascinating and intricate field of study. As we delve into this realm, it calls for further exploration and understanding. Collaboration between athletes, nutritionists, and researchers can pave the way for innovative strategies that leverage the unique properties of magic mushrooms, supporting both performance and overall well-being.

In summary, energy production and muscle growth are complex processes relying on a multifaceted nutritional approach. While a balanced diet is fundamental, strategically using specific nutrients and supplements can enhance athletic performance further. Including magic mushrooms in this equation introduces additional dimensions, potentially providing unique benefits but also requiring careful consideration and expertise. Athletes looking to optimize these aspects of their performance would benefit from personalized guidance from professionals skilled in sports nutrition and familiar with the attributes and interactions of psychedelic substances.

The role of hydration and electrolytes in maintaining peak performance

Hydration and the balance of electrolytes in the body are indispensable in maintaining peak athletic performance. Proper hydration ensures that an athlete's body can perform all its functions efficiently, including temperature regulation, joint lubrication, and nutrient transportation. Electrolytes, such as sodium, potassium, magnesium, and calcium, further contribute to muscle function, nerve transmission, and maintaining the body's acid-base balance.

Athletes lose fluids and electrolytes through sweat during intense training sessions or competitions. If not adequately addressed, this loss can lead to dehydration and electrolyte imbalances, causing fatigue, muscle cramps, decreased coordination, and potentially more severe health issues. Athletes need to replace these losses through a well-planned hydration strategy, considering the quantity of fluid and the quality, including the right balance of electrolytes.

The interplay between magic mushrooms and hydration adds a layer of complexity to this process. As mentioned earlier, the heightened awareness of bodily sensations during a psychedelic experience might influence an athlete's perception of thirst and hydration levels. This altered perception may be a valuable tool, allowing athletes to more precisely tune into their body's needs. However, it also presents a potential risk if misinterpreted, leading to overhydration or underhydration.

Understanding and managing hydration and electrolyte balance within the context of magic mushrooms requires a delicate and individualized approach. Athletes need to be aware of their unique hydration needs, considering factors such as body size, activity level, environmental conditions, and the potential influence of magic mushrooms. Monitoring urine color, tracking weight changes, and paying close attention to how they feel physically are practical ways to ensure they stay hydrated.

The role of hydration and electrolytes in maintaining peak performance is multifaceted and must be considered. When considering using magic mushrooms in conjunction with athletic training, a nuanced and thoughtful approach to hydration strategy is necessary to maximize benefits and minimize risks. The collaboration of sports nutrition professionals, along with ongoing education and self-awareness, can facilitate this process and contribute to enhanced athletic performance.

The impact of magic mushrooms on nutrient absorption and utilization

The interaction of magic mushrooms with nutrient absorption and utilization is a multifaceted topic that extends into various areas of physiological functioning.

Gastrointestinal Impact: Magic mushrooms can distinctly affect the gastrointestinal system, the central hub for nutrient absorption. Some individuals may experience fluctuations in appetite or even digestive discomfort during a macrodosing experience. These changes can affect the digestion and absorption of vital nutrients, including vitamins, minerals, proteins, fats, and carbohydrates. For athletes, an imbalance in nutrient absorption could manifest in altered energy levels, recovery rates, and overall performance, underscoring the need for understanding these interactions.

Metabolic Changes: Beyond the gastrointestinal system, magic mushrooms might shift metabolic pathways responsible for nutrient utilization. Modifying neurotransmitter activity may influence how the body uses energy reserves like glycogen and fatty acids during exercise. This shift in energy expenditure and efficiency in nutrient utilization means that dietary and supplementation strategies may need to be tailored to align with these changes, especially for athletes engaged in rigorous training.

Mind-Body Connection: The enhanced connection between mind and body often reported during a psychedelic experience could offer athletes a more acute awareness of their bodies' nutritional needs and deficiencies. This awareness may lead to more informed and intuitive dietary choices, optimizing nutrient absorption and utilization. However, it should be noted that this connection can vary significantly among individuals and may be interpreted subjectively.

Potential Interactions with Supplements and Medications: The potential interactions between magic mushrooms and certain dietary supplements or medications should be considered. These interactions either amplify or inhibit the absorption and effectiveness of these substances. For example, if an athlete takes supplements that affect serotonin levels, the simultaneous use of magic mushrooms may lead to unexpected physiological outcomes.

In conclusion, the impact of magic mushrooms on nutrient absorption and utilization is complex and requires a nuanced approach. The interplay between magic mushrooms and the body's digestion, metabolism, intuitive awareness, and interactions with other substances presents a rich field for exploration. Understanding and integrating these factors could pave the way for athletes to utilize magic mushrooms to enhance their nutritional strategies, performance, and overall well-being. It highlights the importance of ongoing research and personalized approaches to unlock the potential benefits of athletic enhancement.

The Importance of a Personalized Approach

When combining magic mushrooms with other performance enhancers, it is crucial to recognize that each individual is unique and will respond differently to various substances and combinations. A personalized approach allows athletes to tailor their regimen to their specific needs, goals, and individual responses, maximizing the potential benefits and minimizing risks.

Assessing individual needs and goals to determine the optimal combination of enhancers: Understanding your athletic goals, current performance levels, and individual needs is the first step in developing a personalized approach to combining magic mushrooms with other performance enhancers. By evaluating these factors, you can determine the most suitable substances and dosages to support your objectives while minimizing the risk of adverse effects.

Monitoring and adjusting combinations based on personal experiences and results: As you experiment with different combinations of performance enhancers, it is crucial to closely monitor your experiences, results, and any potential side effects. This information will help you fine-tune your regimen, making adjustments as necessary to optimize your performance while ensuring safety and well-being.

The role of genetic factors and individual variability in response to performance enhancers: Genetic factors can influence how individuals respond to specific performance enhancers, including magic mushrooms. These differences can impact the effectiveness and safety of certain substances or combinations. Considering your unique genetic makeup and individual variability, you can develop a more tailored and practical approach to combining magic mushrooms with other performance-enhancing substances.

Seeking guidance from professionals and experts in sports performance and nutrition: Consulting with healthcare professionals, sports nutritionists, or performance coaches experienced in using psychedelics and other performance enhancers can provide valuable guidance in developing a personalized approach. These experts can offer insights into the most effective combinations and dosages based on your individual needs, goals, and circumstances, as well as provide support in monitoring your progress and adjusting your regimen as needed.

In conclusion, a personalized approach to combining magic mushrooms with other performance enhancers is essential for achieving optimal results while maintaining safety and well-being. By understanding your needs and goals, monitoring your experiences and results, and seeking professional guidance, you can develop a tailored regimen that best supports your athletic performance and personal growth.

Synergistic Effects of Magic Mushrooms with Other Performance-Enhancing Substances

The intriguing world of performance-enhancing substances and their potential synergistic effects with magic mushrooms offers athletes new avenues for improving their performance. Combining different substances can sometimes yield powerful results, but it's crucial to understand the benefits and potential risks of these combinations and the legal and ethical implications involved.

This exploration covers legal and illegal performance-enhancing substances that athletes may consider using with magic mushrooms. We will delve into the mechanisms by which these substances can potentially enhance physical and mental performance and how they may interact with the psychedelic compounds found in magic mushrooms. Additionally, we will discuss the importance of thoroughly researching and understanding the potential side effects, interactions, and risks associated with combining these substances. Athletes need to prioritize their health and well-being while striving for peak performance, and this can be achieved by making informed decisions regarding the use of performance-enhancing substances.

Moreover, we will examine the ethical considerations surrounding the use of banned substances in competitive sports and athletes' responsibility to maintain the integrity of their chosen field. Balancing the desire for improved performance with the need for fair competition is a crucial aspect of any athlete's journey.

Finally, we will emphasize the necessity for further research in this field, as it has the potential to unlock new ways of maximizing human potential in sports and other high-performance endeavors. This could ultimately lead to groundbreaking advancements in understanding human performance optimization and developing novel strategies for athletes to achieve their goals safely and effectively.

Legal Performance-Enhancing Substances

Beta-alanine: Beta-alanine is a naturally occurring, non-essential amino acid that has garnered significant attention in sports performance. Its primary function serves as a precursor for carnosine, a dipeptide that acts as a buffer against muscle fatigue and supports endurance.

BCAAs (Branched-chain amino acids): BCAAs are essential amino acids that include leucine, isoleucine, and valine. They are critical for muscle growth, recovery, and endurance. BCAAs can be found in many protein-rich foods and are commonly taken as supplements to support athletic performance.

L-citrulline: L-citrulline is an amino acid shown to improve blood flow and oxygen delivery to muscles, which can enhance overall athletic performance. It is often taken as a supplement to support cardiovascular health and may be particularly beneficial for endurance athletes.

Pre-workout supplements: Pre-workout supplements are designed to boost energy, focus, and endurance during workouts. They typically contain a combination of ingredients such as caffeine, amino acids, and other performance-enhancing compounds. These supplements can help athletes maximize their training sessions and improve overall performance.

Creatine: Creatine is a well-researched and widely used performance-enhancing supplement that helps increase muscle strength, power, and size. It works by increasing the availability of creatine phosphate, an energy source for quick, high-intensity muscle contractions. Creatine supplementation is particularly beneficial for athletes involved in strength and power sports.

Nitric oxide boosters: Nitric oxide boosters are supplements that help increase nitric oxide levels in the body, leading to improved blood flow and oxygen delivery to working muscles. This can enhance endurance, muscle pump, and overall athletic performance. Common ingredients in nitric oxide boosters include arginine, citrulline, and beetroot extract.

Caffeine: Caffeine is a widely consumed stimulant that can enhance athletic performance by increasing alertness, focus, and energy levels. It has been shown to improve endurance, reduce the perception of effort, and even increase strength in some individuals. Caffeine is commonly found in pre-workout supplements, energy drinks, and coffee.

Sodium bicarbonate: Sodium bicarbonate, also known as baking soda, is an alkaline substance that can help buffer lactic acid buildup in the muscles during high-intensity exercise. This buffering effect can delay the onset of muscle fatigue, improve anaerobic capacity, and enhance overall performance in sports that involve short, intense bursts of activity.

Carnitine: Carnitine is a compound that plays a crucial role in transporting fatty acids into the mitochondria, where they are used to produce energy. Supplementing with carnitine may improve endurance by enhancing fat utilization, sparing glycogen stores, and reducing lactic acid buildup during exercise.

Taurine: Taurine is an amino acid that supports various aspects of athletic performance, including muscle function, hydration, and electrolyte balance. It is commonly found in energy drinks and pre-workout supplements, and it may help reduce muscle cramps, improve exercise capacity, and enhance recovery.

Glutamine: Glutamine is the most abundant amino acid in the human body and plays a vital role in immune function, gut health, and muscle recovery. Athletes often supplement with glutamine to help maintain muscle mass, reduce muscle soreness, and support overall recovery during intense training or competition periods.

Nitrate: Nitrate is a naturally occurring compound found in vegetables like beets and spinach, which can be converted into nitric oxide in the body. Nitric oxide is a vasodilator that helps widen blood vessels, improving blood flow and oxygen delivery to the muscles. Supplementing with nitrate, or consuming nitrate-rich foods, may improve endurance, reduce oxygen consumption during exercise, and increase overall performance.

HMB (Beta-hydroxy-beta-methylbutyrate): HMB is a metabolite of the amino acid leucine, which has been shown to promote muscle growth, strength, and recovery. Supplementing with HMB may help prevent muscle breakdown, reduce exercise-induced muscle damage, and enhance overall strength and endurance sports performance. HMB may help athletes increase lean muscle mass, enhance recovery, and improve overall performance, particularly during high-intensity workouts.

Betaine: Betaine is a compound found in foods like spinach and beets, and it has been shown to support athletic performance by enhancing muscle power, strength, and endurance. It also helps reduce inflammation and oxidative stress, benefiting recovery and overall health.

Cordyceps: Cordyceps is a fungus used in traditional Chinese medicine for centuries to promote energy, endurance, and overall health. Recent research suggests that cordyceps improve athletic performance by increasing oxygen utilization, enhancing energy production, and reducing fatigue.

Beetroot Extract: Beetroot extract has gained popularity among athletes due to its high nitrate content. Nitrates can be converted into nitric oxide, which may help improve blood flow, oxygen delivery to muscles, and overall athletic performance. Supplementing with beetroot extract has been shown to enhance endurance, increase time to exhaustion, and improve exercise efficiency.

Agmatine: Agmatine is a naturally occurring compound derived from the amino acid L-arginine. It has potential benefits for athletes due to its ability to modulate nitric oxide synthesis, which can improve blood flow and oxygen delivery to muscles. Agmatine supplementation enhances endurance, reduces muscle fatigue, and promotes faster recovery after intense workouts. Additionally, agmatine has been suggested to possess pain-relieving and neuroprotective properties, which could further support athletic performance and recovery.

Supplementation Regimen Examples

It's important to note that individual responses to supplements and microdosing may vary, and it's essential to consult with a healthcare professional, sports nutritionist, or trainer before starting any new supplement regimen. However, here is a general outline of how you might incorporate these supplements along with microdosing psilocybin:

Pre-workout:

1. Caffeine (100-200mg): For increased energy and focus. Take 30-60 minutes before exercise.
2. Beta-alanine (2-5g): For enhanced endurance and reduced muscle fatigue. Take 30 minutes before exercise.
3. L-citrulline (6-8g): For improved blood flow and oxygen delivery to muscles. Take 30-60 minutes before exercise.

4. Taurine (1-2g): For improved muscle function and reduced oxidative stress. Take 30-60 minutes before exercise.

Performance Enhancement:

1. Microdosing psilocybin: Typically 1/10th to 1/20th of a regular dose (0.1-0.3g dried mushrooms or equivalent). Take on a schedule such as one day on, two days off, or every third day. Adjust the schedule based on individual responses and needs.
2. BCAAs (5-10g): For muscle growth, recovery, and endurance. Consume during or after exercise.
3. Creatine (5g daily): For increased strength and power. It can be taken at any time during the day, but many athletes prefer to take it post-workout.

Recovery:

1. Protein powder (20-40g): For muscle repair and growth. Consume within 30 minutes of completing your workout.
2. HMB (3g): For muscle recovery and reduced muscle breakdown. Consume post-workout.
3. Ashwagandha or Rhodiola (dosage as per manufacturer's recommendation): For stress management and recovery. Take in the morning or evening, as per individual preference.

It's crucial to start with the lowest recommended dosages and gradually increase as needed, based on individual response and tolerance. Remember that this is just a general outline; personalizing your supplement regimen based on your specific needs and goals is essential.

Here's an example of a supplement regimen tailored for strength training, incorporating microdosing psilocybin:

Pre-workout:

1. Caffeine (100-200mg): For increased energy and focus. Take 30-60 minutes before exercise.
2. Beta-alanine (2-5g): For enhanced endurance and reduced muscle fatigue. Take 30 minutes before exercise.
3. Creatine (5g): For increased strength and power. It can be taken pre-workout or post-workout, depending on individual preference.

Performance Enhancement:

1. Microdosing psilocybin: Typically 1/10th to 1/20th of a regular dose (0.1-0.3g dried mushrooms or equivalent). Take on a schedule such as one day on, two days off, or every third day. Adjust the schedule based on individual responses and needs.
2. BCAAs (5-10g): For muscle growth, recovery, and endurance. Consume during or after exercise.
3. L-carnitine (1-3g): For improved fat metabolism and energy production. Take 30-60 minutes before exercise.

Competitions:

1. Sodium bicarbonate (0.3g/kg body weight): Sodium bicarbonate, also known as baking soda, can help buffer lactic acid build-up and delay fatigue during high-intensity strength training events. Take it 60-90 minutes before the competition, preferably with a carbohydrate-rich meal.
2. Beetroot juice (6-8mmol nitrate): Beetroot juice contains nitrate, which may improve blood flow and oxygen

delivery to the muscles, enhancing performance in strength training competitions. Consume 6-8mmol nitrate (around 500ml of beetroot juice) 2-3 hours before the event.

3. Vasodilators: Supplements like L-arginine or L-citrulline can enhance blood flow and muscle nutrient delivery, potentially boosting performance in strength-based competitions. Take these supplements 30-60 minutes before the event, following the recommended dosages.

4. Mental preparation: Mental preparation techniques such as visualization, goal setting, and positive self-talk can help athletes stay focused and confident during strength training competitions.

5. Optimal warm-up: Engage in an effective warm-up routine to increase muscle temperature, blood flow, and joint mobility, preparing the body for optimal performance in strength-based events.

6. Intra-competition nutrition: Depending on the duration of the competition, consume easily digestible carbohydrates (e.g., sports drinks, gels, or bars) and fluids to maintain energy levels and hydration.

7. Proper rest and recovery: Ensure adequate rest between training sessions leading up to the competition and between competition events, allowing muscles to recover and minimizing the risk of injury.

8. Tapering: Reducing training volume and intensity a week or two before the competition can help minimize fatigue while maintaining performance gains.

Recovery:

1. Protein powder (20-40g): For muscle repair and growth. Consume within 30 minutes of completing your workout.

2. HMB (3g): For muscle recovery and reduced muscle breakdown. Consume post-workout.

3. Taurine (1-2g): For improved muscle function and reduced oxidative stress. Take post-workout.

4. Omega-3 fatty acids (1-3g): For reduced inflammation and improved recovery. Consume with a meal, once per day.

Remember that this is just a general outline; personalizing your supplement regimen based on your specific needs and goals is essential. Start with the lowest recommended dosages and gradually increase as needed, based on individual response and tolerance. Always consult a professional before starting any new supplement routine, especially when combining substances like magic mushrooms with other supplements.

Endurance Race Example

Here's an example of a supplement regimen tailored for endurance races, incorporating microdosing psilocybin:

Pre-workout:

1. Caffeine (100-200mg): For increased energy and focus. Take 30-60 minutes before exercise.
2. L-citrulline (6-8g): For improved blood flow and oxygen delivery to muscles. Take 30-60 minutes before exercise.
3. Beta-alanine (2-5g): For enhanced endurance and reduced muscle fatigue. Take 30 minutes before exercise.

Performance Enhancement:

1. Microdosing psilocybin: Typically 1/10th to 1/20th of a regular dose (0.1-0.3g dried mushrooms or equivalent). Take on a schedule such as one day on, two days off, or every third day. Adjust the schedule based on individual responses and needs.
2. BCAAs (5-10g): For muscle growth, recovery, and endurance. Consume during or after exercise.
3. Cordyceps (1-3g): For increased oxygen utilization and energy production. Take 30-60 minutes before exercise.

During Race:

1. Electrolytes: Endurance races can lead to significant loss of electrolytes (sodium, potassium, magnesium, and calcium) through sweat. Consuming electrolyte supplements or sports drinks can help replenish these essential minerals and prevent cramps, dehydration, and imbalances.
2. Slow-release carbohydrates: For longer endurance races, consuming slow-release carbohydrates such as energy bars, oatmeal, or whole-grain bread can help maintain steady energy levels by providing a sustained source of glucose.
3. Caffeine (3-6mg/kg body weight): Caffeine can be an effective performance enhancer for endurance athletes by increasing alertness and reducing perceived exertion. Consume caffeine 30-60 minutes before the race or in divided doses during the event, depending on individual tolerance.
4. Glutamine (5-10g): Glutamine can help support immune function and muscle recovery during endurance events. Mix it with water or an electrolyte drink and sip it throughout the race.
5. Antioxidants: Endurance races can generate oxidative stress due to prolonged physical exertion. Consuming antioxidant-rich foods or supplements such as vitamin C, E, or polyphenols (found in berries, green tea, and dark chocolate) may help protect against cellular damage and support recovery.
6. Adaptogens: Adaptogenic herbs such as Rhodiola rosea or Siberian ginseng can help improve endurance, reduce fatigue, and support the body's stress response during prolonged events.
7. Proper pacing: Monitoring your pace and heart rate can help you maintain a sustainable intensity level

throughout the endurance race, preventing burnout and optimizing performance.

8. Fueling strategy: Develop a fueling strategy that includes regular intake of carbohydrates, electrolytes, and fluids, adjusting based on the race duration, climate, and individual needs.

Recovery:

1. Protein powder (20-40g): For muscle repair and growth. Consume within 30 minutes of completing your workout or race.
2. Taurine (1-2g): For improved muscle function and reduced oxidative stress. Take post-workout or post-race.
3. Omega-3 fatty acids (1-3g): For reduced inflammation and improved recovery. Consume with a meal, once per day.

Remember that this is just a general outline; personalizing your supplement regimen based on your specific needs and goals is essential. Start with the lowest recommended dosages and gradually increase as needed, based on individual response and tolerance. Always consult a professional before starting any new supplement routine, especially when combining substances like magic mushrooms with other supplements.

Brazilian Jiu-Jitsu (BJJ) Competition Example

Here's an example of a supplement regimen tailored for a Brazilian Jiu-Jitsu (BJJ) competition, incorporating microdosing psilocybin:

Pre-workout/Pre-competition:

1. Caffeine (100-200mg): For increased energy and focus. Take 30-60 minutes before exercise or competition.

2. L-tyrosine (500-2000mg): For improved focus and stress resistance. Take 30-60 minutes before exercise or competition.
3. Cordyceps (1-3g): For increased oxygen utilization and energy production. Take 30-60 minutes before exercise or competition.

Performance Enhancement:

1. Microdosing psilocybin: Typically 1/10th to 1/20th of a regular dose (0.1-0.3g dried mushrooms or equivalent). Take on a schedule such as one day on, two days off, or every third day. Adjust the schedule based on individual responses and needs.
2. BCAAs (5-10g): For muscle growth, recovery, and endurance. Consume during or after exercise or competition.
3. Creatine (3-5g daily): For increased strength and power output. Take daily, with or without a loading phase.

During Competition:

1. Electrolyte supplement: For maintaining hydration and electrolyte balance during the competition. Consume according to the product's recommended dosage and instructions.
2. Carbohydrate gels or chews: For maintaining energy levels during the competition. Consume as needed based on personal preference and competition duration.
3. Mental techniques: Utilize techniques such as visualization, mindfulness, and positive self-talk to maintain focus and stay calm under pressure.
4. Breathing exercises: Practice deep, controlled breathing to help manage stress and anxiety levels and promote relaxation and focus.
5. Beta-alanine (3-6g daily): For increased endurance and reduced muscle fatigue. It can be taken as a pre-workout

supplement, or split into smaller doses throughout the day to reduce the risk of experiencing a tingling sensation (paresthesia).

6. Citrulline malate (6-8g): For improved blood flow and oxygen delivery to muscles. Take 30-60 minutes before exercise or competition.

7. Fast-acting carbohydrates: Simple carbohydrates like sports drinks, fruits, or energy gels can provide quick energy during competition, helping to maintain glycogen stores and prevent energy crashes.

8. Intra-workout BCAAs or EAA supplements: Consuming branched-chain amino acids (BCAAs) or essential amino acids (EAAs) during competition can help maintain energy levels, promote muscle recovery, and reduce fatigue.

9. Adequate hydration: Proper hydration is crucial during competition. Drink water consistently, aiming for small sips every 15-20 minutes, depending on the intensity and duration of the competition.

10. Cooling strategies: Use cooling techniques such as ice packs, cold towels, or even a cool water mist to manage body temperature and prevent overheating during intense competitions.

Recovery:

1. Protein powder (20-40g): For muscle repair and growth. Consume within 30 minutes of completing your workout or competition.

2. Taurine (1-2g): For improved muscle function and reduced oxidative stress. Take post-workout or post-competition.

3. Omega-3 fatty acids (1-3g): For reduced inflammation and improved recovery. Consume with a meal, once per day.

Remember that this is just a general outline; personalizing your supplement regimen based on your specific needs and goals is essential. Start with the lowest recommended dosages and gradually increase as needed, based on individual response and tolerance. Always consult a professional before starting any new supplement routine, especially when combining substances like magic mushrooms with other supplements.

As with any new supplement or strategy, testing them during training is essential to understand how your body responds and make any necessary adjustments. Consult a professional before starting any new supplement routine or performance-enhancing strategy.

Illegal Performance-Enhancing Substances

It is important to note that the use of illegal performance-enhancing substances carries significant risks, including health issues, ethical concerns, and potential disqualification from competitions or bans from sports organizations. However, for the sake of understanding, here is a list of some illegal substances that athletes have used to enhance performance:

Anabolic steroids: These synthetic hormones mimic testosterone's effects, promoting muscle growth, strength, and recovery. They come with significant health risks like liver damage, cardiovascular issues, hormonal imbalances, and psychological effects.

(HGH) Human growth hormone: HGH is a hormone that may increase muscle mass and improve recovery. It is banned in professional sports due to potential health risks, including joint pain, swelling, insulin resistance, and an increased cancer risk.

EPO (Erythropoietin): EPO is a hormone that stimulates red blood cell production, enhancing oxygen delivery to muscles. It is banned in professional sports due to the risk of blood clotting, stroke, heart attack, and other serious side effects.

(SARMs) Selective Androgen Receptor Modulators: SARMs selectively bind to androgen receptors, promoting muscle growth and fat loss without many side effects associated with anabolic steroids. They are currently unapproved for human use and banned in professional sports.

Blood doping: Blood doping involves either the infusion of an athlete's blood or a donor's blood to increase red blood cell count and oxygen-carrying capacity, enhancing endurance. This practice is illegal and poses significant health risks, such as blood clotting, infections, and cardiovascular issues.

Amphetamines: Amphetamines are stimulants that can enhance alertness, focus, and energy levels. They are illegal in sports due to their potential for addiction, cardiovascular complications, and other serious health risks.

Diuretics: Diuretics are substances that increase urine production, causing rapid weight loss, and are sometimes used by athletes to meet weight requirements in specific sports categories. They are banned in professional sports due to the risk of dehydration, electrolyte imbalances, and kidney damage.

Beta-2 agonists: These substances, typically used to treat asthma, can stimulate the nervous system and increase aerobic capacity, strength, and endurance. They are banned in professional sports because they can cause side effects like heart palpitations, tremors, and rapid heart rate.

Insulin: Although primarily used to manage diabetes, some athletes may misuse insulin to enhance muscle growth and recovery by increasing glucose and amino acid uptake in muscle cells. Insulin abuse is dangerous and can lead to hypoglycemia, seizures, coma, or even death.

Prohormones: Prohormones are precursors to anabolic steroids that can convert to active hormones. They are used by some athletes to increase muscle mass and strength but are banned in professional sports. They can cause similar side effects as anabolic steroids, such as liver toxicity, hormonal imbalances, and cardiovascular issues.

Designer steroids: Designer steroids are chemically modified versions of anabolic steroids that are created to evade detection by anti-doping tests. They are illegal and can carry similar health risks as traditional anabolic steroids.

Stimulants (other than amphetamines): Other stimulants, like ephedrine and methylhexanamine, can increase alertness, focus, and energy. They are banned in professional sports due to their potential for addiction, cardiovascular complications, and other serious health risks.

Peptide hormones: Some athletes use peptide hormones like IGF-1, CJC-1295, and GHRP-6 to boost growth hormone levels, which can improve muscle mass and recovery. These substances are banned in professional sports and can lead to potential health risks, including joint pain, swelling, and an increased cancer risk.

Masking agents: Masking agents are substances used to hide the presence of performance-enhancing drugs in drug tests. They include substances like epitestosterone, probenecid, and plasma expanders. These agents are banned in professional sports due to their potential to undermine the integrity of anti-doping efforts and may also carry health risks.

S-23: S-23 is a non-steroidal selective androgen receptor modulator (SARM) currently being researched for potential medical applications. Some athletes use it for muscle growth, fat loss, and increased bone density. However, it is unapproved for human use and banned in professional sports. The long-term effects and safety profile of S-23 need to be better understood.

Again, it is crucial to emphasize that using illegal performance-enhancing substances is not recommended and carries significant risks for the athlete's health and their standing within the sports community. Always prioritize safe and legal methods for improving performance and consult with professionals for guidance.

Disclaimer: The information provided in this text is intended for informational and educational purposes only and is not meant to be taken as medical advice. Please consult with a qualified healthcare professional before making any decisions regarding using performance-enhancing substances or any other supplements mentioned. Illegal performance-enhancing substances are not endorsed or recommended, and athletes should always adhere to the rules and regulations of their respective sports governing bodies. Individual results may vary, and proper training, nutrition, and recovery are crucial components of a well-rounded athletic program.

Potential Risks and Ethical Considerations

As we delve into the world of performance enhancement through magic mushrooms and other substances, it is crucial to address the potential risks and ethical considerations associated with these practices. This part of our discussion will explore the health risks and side effects of combining magic mushrooms with other performance enhancers and the ethical implications of using banned substances in competitive sports. Additionally, we will highlight the necessity of further research to understand better these combinations' safety, efficacy, and long-term consequences. By examining these essential topics, we aim to promote responsible and informed use of performance-enhancing substances, ensuring that athletes and fitness enthusiasts prioritize their health and well-being while pursuing their goals.

Understanding Health Risks and Side Effects

The pursuit of optimal athletic performance often leads athletes to explore various combinations of substances, including magic mushrooms. While synergistic effects may offer unique benefits, they can also present significant health risks and side effects. It is vital to approach these combinations cautiously, beginning with low doses and closely observing one's physical and mental state.

Short-term risks and side effects may vary from mild physical reactions, such as nausea, dizziness, headaches, and dehydration, to more severe issues like heart palpitations and increased blood pressure. These short-term effects could significantly impair an athlete's immediate performance, affecting coordination, focus, endurance, and decision-making abilities. Psychological responses like anxiety, confusion, or paranoia might also emerge, impacting immediate well-being and possibly leading to long-term mental health problems.

The long-term risks and health implications add another layer of complexity to the synergistic use of magic mushrooms with other substances. Prolonged use of specific combinations may damage vital organs, such as the liver, kidneys, or heart, especially concerning substances metabolized or filtered through these organs. Interactions with hormonal supplements could create imbalances that affect everything from muscle growth to mood regulation. Moreover, the risk of developing chronic health conditions, including cardiovascular diseases or neurological disorders, might increase with long-term exposure.

Understanding these risks requires careful research, consultation with healthcare providers, and collaboration with sports nutritionists or pharmacologists. Knowledge of the pharmacodynamics and pharmacokinetics of each substance, coupled with their potential interactions, is essential to minimize risks. Continuous monitoring and willingness to make adjustments, starting with low doses and gradually modifying them based on personal experiences and professional guidance, can help find an optimal balance without compromising health.

Athletes must weigh the potential benefits against the known risks when considering the synergistic use of magic mushrooms and other performance enhancers. This area, filled with potential rewards and significant risks, demands an approach rooted in scientific understanding, caution, and a profound commitment to overall well-being. By considering short-term and long-term effects, athletes can make more informed and responsible decisions about their performance strategies.

Ethical Implications

Pursuing excellence in sports often leads athletes to explore various means of enhancing their performance. While training, nutrition, and legitimate supplementation form the core of this pursuit, the use of banned substances often lurks at the fringes. Combining magic mushrooms and other performance enhancers with competitive sports raises significant ethical considerations that demand careful reflection.

The landscape of competitive sports is governed by a complex web of rules and regulations, some of which explicitly forbid the use of certain substances. Depending on the jurisdiction and sporting body, magic mushrooms, classified as psychedelics, may fall into this category. The temptation to use these substances to gain an edge must be weighed against the ethical obligations to adhere to the rules of the sport, the expectations of fair play, and the potential consequences of a ban or other penalties.

Further complicating the ethical landscape is the broader question of fairness and integrity in sports competitions. While using magic mushrooms and other enhancers might be seen as innovative or cutting-edge by some, others argue that it violates the principles of a level playing field. This raises fundamental questions about what constitutes fair competition and how far athletes can achieve victory. These questions are not quickly answered, and the lines can blur, but they lie at the heart of the ongoing debate about using performance-enhancing substances in sports. Balancing personal ambition with a commitment to the shared values of sportsmanship requires careful thought and a clear understanding of the sport's rules and one's own ethical principles.

Necessity of Further Research

While anecdotal evidence suggests that some combinations of magic mushrooms and other performance-enhancing substances may yield beneficial effects, the scientific understanding of these synergistic effects still needs to be improved. More research is needed to evaluate the safety, efficacy, and optimal dosages for these combinations and uncover potential new combinations that may further enhance athletic performance. This research should be conducted in controlled, ethical environments prioritizing participant safety and informed consent.

As more athletes and researchers explore the potential benefits of combining magic mushrooms with other performance-enhancing substances, it is essential to gather data on the safety and efficacy of these combinations. Conducting clinical trials and observational studies will help establish a more robust understanding of these combinations' potential risks and benefits, allowing athletes to make informed decisions about their use. This knowledge can also guide sports organizations in updating their regulations and guidelines to reflect the current state of scientific understanding better.

Developing Guidelines for Responsible Use and Education

As we better understand the synergistic effects of magic mushrooms and other performance-enhancing substances, it is crucial to develop evidence-based recommendations to guide athletes and fitness enthusiasts in their quest for improved performance. These guidelines should consider the unique needs and goals of individuals and the specific substances being combined. By offering clear and well-researched recommendations, we can ensure that those seeking performance enhancement do so in a safe and effective manner.

Alongside developing guidelines for responsible use, promoting education and awareness about the potential risks and benefits of combining magic mushrooms with other performance enhancers is essential. This includes making information readily available to athletes, coaches, and other individuals involved in sports and fitness. Educational resources should cover topics such as responsible dosing, potential side effects, and strategies for mitigating risks. By fostering a culture of informed decision-making, we can empower athletes to make choices that align with their goals while prioritizing their health and well-being.

Finally, promoting open dialogue and collaboration among athletes, coaches, researchers, and other stakeholders is critical to advancing our understanding of the synergistic effects of magic mushrooms and other performance enhancers. By encouraging the sharing of experiences, research findings, and best practices, we can create a supportive community that fosters responsible use and ongoing exploration of these substances. This collaborative approach will ultimately lead to better outcomes for athletes and the broader sports community and contribute to a greater understanding of the potential applications of these substances in the pursuit of enhanced performance.

Emphasizing Responsible Use and Encouraging Further Research

It is essential to emphasize the importance of responsible use when combining magic mushrooms with other performance-enhancing substances. Athletes and fitness enthusiasts should prioritize their health and well-being, making informed decisions based on evidence, guidelines, and personal experiences. By being mindful of potential risks and side effects, individuals can minimize harm while maximizing the potential benefits of these combinations.

Given the limited body of research currently available on the synergistic effects of magic mushrooms and other performance enhancers, there is a pressing need for further investigation in this area. Future studies should explore the safety, efficacy, and long-term consequences of combining these substances, focusing on understanding individual variability and potential interactions. This research will ultimately contribute to developing evidence-based recommendations and educational resources, ensuring athletes and fitness enthusiasts can make informed decisions about their performance-enhancement strategies.

As our understanding of the potential synergistic effects of magic mushrooms and other performance enhancers grows, we must remain open to new possibilities and discoveries. By fostering a culture of curiosity, collaboration, and learning, we can pave the way for novel performance-enhancement approaches prioritizing safety and effectiveness. In doing so, we can support athletes and fitness enthusiasts in pursuing excellence while contributing to the broader scientific understanding of these powerful substances and their potential applications in sports and beyond.

Mindfulness Practices for Athletic Performance

As athletes continually strive to push their limits and achieve peak performance, mindfulness practices have become a powerful tool to complement physical training. By harnessing the power of meditation, visualization, breathwork, and movement-based practices such as yoga, individuals can develop more significant focus, resilience, and self-awareness, ultimately contributing to their overall athletic performance. In this chapter, we will explore the various mindfulness techniques and their applications in sports and fitness, examining how they can enhance athletic abilities and promote injury prevention and rehabilitation. By incorporating these practices into their daily routines, athletes can cultivate a holistic approach to their performance, nurturing both the body and the mind.

The Power of Meditation and Visualization

Meditation and visualization are two closely related practices with immense potential for athletes seeking to elevate their performance. These methods have been embraced across various sports disciplines due to their substantial mental and physical benefits.

Meditation, which involves training the mind to be present and focused, can enhance an athlete's concentration, reduce stress, and improve emotional regulation. Traditional meditation techniques like mindfulness encourage a non-judgmental awareness of the present moment. By regularly engaging in meditation, athletes can learn to maintain a calm and composed demeanor, even under high-pressure situations. The physiological benefits include lower heart rate and blood pressure, aiding recovery and overall well-being. This steadiness and presence of mind translate into an ability to perform at their best when stakes are high.

Conversely, visualization is a mental rehearsal technique that involves creating vivid mental images of specific athletic feats, outcomes, or scenarios. Whether visualizing the perfect free-throw shot in basketball or a flawless execution of a gymnastic routine, the process engages the same neural pathways involved in physical performance. By repeatedly visualizing themselves executing a particular movement or achieving a desired outcome, athletes can develop greater confidence and a stronger mind-body connection. This mental rehearsal primes the brain and body for action, making it more likely that the athlete will execute the envisioned performance when it truly matters.

The combination of meditation and visualization can be especially powerful. Meditation lays the groundwork for effective visualization by cultivating a focused and receptive mental state. Athletes can use meditation to center themselves and then proceed to visualization exercises, maximizing the impact of their mental rehearsal.

Both meditation and visualization can be practiced independently or integrated into an athlete's daily routine. They don't require any special equipment or facilities, making them accessible to athletes at all levels. With consistent practice, these techniques can contribute to improved athletic performance and foster a greater sense of well-being and mental resilience.

Coaches and sports psychologists are increasingly recognizing these practices as integral to modern sports training. The positive effects extend beyond the playing field into personal development, enhancing self-awareness, empathy, and overall life satisfaction. By investing in cultivating these mental skills, athletes are not only sharpening their competitive edge but enriching their lives and laying a foundation for long-term success both in their sport and life.

Breathwork for Enhanced Focus and Recovery: The Unsung Hero of Athletic Mindfulness

Breathwork is a powerful yet often overlooked tool in the athlete's mindfulness arsenal. Aside from being a mere physiological necessity, conscious breath control is a conduit for enhanced athletic performance and faster recovery. The practice of breathwork doesn't just involve inhaling and exhaling; it's a nuanced technique requiring mindfulness and intent.

When delving into the realm of breathwork, it's evident that the practice is not monolithic; it's a spectrum of techniques designed to serve many needs and scenarios athletes may encounter. Let's unpack some of the prominent methodologies to understand their unique advantages.

Starting with the most accessible, deep breathing exercises serve as the foundational building blocks of breathwork. These techniques often involve inhaling deeply through the nose, holding the breath momentarily, and then exhaling fully through the mouth. Simple yet effective, deep breathing can activate the body's relaxation response, making it ideal for athletes needing to de-stress quickly before or after an event. It is also invaluable for enhancing the oxygenation of the muscles, which can be beneficial during both anaerobic and aerobic exertion.

Pranayama, originating from the yoga tradition, introduces an element of discipline and structure to breath control. Often integrated into yoga routines, pranayama techniques like 'Nadi Shodhana' (alternate nostril breathing) and 'Ujjayi' (victorious breath) can help athletes gain better control over their physiological responses. For instance, Nadi Shodhana is known to balance the body's energy flow and induce calmness, making it suitable for pre-competition mental preparation. On the other hand, Ujjayi creates a soothing sound that can serve as a focal point, allowing athletes to concentrate better during performance.

The Wim Hof Method has gained widespread recognition for its almost superhuman claims—increased stress resilience, enhanced immune function, and even the ability to withstand extreme cold temperatures. Combining specific breathing patterns with cold exposure and meditation teaches athletes how to tap into their autonomic nervous system. The practice has been widespread among endurance athletes for improving mental fortitude and physical stamina.

Holotropic Breathwork is a more intense, session-based approach often facilitated by certified practitioners. While not for everyone, this technique aims to induce altered states of consciousness, providing deeper insights into one's psychological makeup. Some athletes have reported experiences of profound self-discovery that translated into improved mental resilience and focus in their athletic pursuits.

The diverse methods within breathwork offer tailored solutions for specific needs—calming an overactive mind, enhancing focus, boosting energy, or gaining a deeper understanding of oneself. Athletes willing to explore these varied techniques will likely find keys to unlock new dimensions of both their physical and mental potential.

Breathwork's unparalleled capacity to manage stress is one of its most vital contributions to athletic performance. When an athlete is in the heat of competition or navigating the rigors of intense training, the stress response—commonly known as the 'fight or flight' mechanism—can be activated. Elevated heart rate, quickened breath, and adrenaline rush are all physiological changes that can either make or break a performance. This is where breathwork becomes invaluable; it acts like a dial on this stress response system, allowing athletes to fine-tune their physiological state.

One of the most immediate benefits of controlled breathing in stressful situations is its impact on heart rate regulation. An elevated heart rate can result in jitteriness, reduced fine motor control, and impaired decision-making—none of which are conducive to peak performance. Techniques that focus on elongated exhales, for instance, can stimulate the vagus nerve, lowering heart rate and blood pressure. Athletes can employ this strategy just before a critical moment in the competition, such as a penalty kick or a free throw, to maintain composure and increase the likelihood of successful execution.

Additionally, breathwork can directly affect the adrenal system, which releases hormones like cortisol and adrenaline during stress. Certain breathwork practices help create a more balanced hormonal environment, reducing the adverse effects of stress hormones while retaining enough for enhanced responsiveness and alertness. This delicate balance is crucial for athletes in sports that require quick decision-making under pressure, such as basketball, soccer, or martial arts.

Another overlooked advantage of breathwork is its role in combating fatigue. Muscles need oxygen for optimal performance, and targeted breathing techniques can ensure more efficient oxygen delivery to muscle tissue. This can delay the onset of fatigue and improve endurance and power output, giving athletes a critical edge in long-duration events like marathons, triathlons, or multi-set matches.

Breathwork also excels in its ability to improve focus and drown out distractions. Distractions are a constant obstacle to peak performance, whether it's the roars of a crowd, the tension of a high-stakes moment, or even self-imposed pressure and expectations. Specific breath-focused techniques can serve as an anchoring point, allowing athletes to center their attention effectively. In a way, it offers a mental shield, insulating them from external noise and internal chatter.

Breathwork provides a versatile toolkit for immediate physiological and psychological adjustment. It enables athletes to manage stress effectively, creating optimal internal conditions for peak performance. Whether it's to calm frayed nerves, maintain razor-sharp focus, or stave off encroaching fatigue, breathwork emerges as a real-time strategy with far-reaching implications for athletic excellence.

Breathwork's application extends far beyond the immediacy of performance, offering benefits in the crucial but often neglected area of post-performance recovery. The role of the parasympathetic nervous system—often called the "rest and digest" system—becomes crucial here. High-level athletic exertion stresses both the muscular and central nervous systems, leading to a condition known as 'sympathetic dominance,' where the body's stress systems are in an ongoing state of alertness. This state is counterproductive for recovery. By consciously manipulating the breath, athletes can engage the parasympathetic system, effectively switching gears from a state of high alert to one of rest and recovery.

Engaging the parasympathetic system through deep, controlled breathing techniques can have a cascading effect on various physiological parameters that are critical to recovery. One of the most immediate outcomes is improved sleep quality. Sleep is a cornerstone of effective recovery; it's the period where the body undergoes most of its repair and regeneration processes. Poor or inadequate sleep can impair muscle recovery, decrease cognitive function, and increase injury susceptibility. By utilizing breathwork to induce relaxation and potentially enhance sleep quality, athletes set the stage for more efficient muscle repair and mental rejuvenation.

Another notable benefit lies in the anti-inflammatory effects of breathwork. Inflammation is a double-edged sword in athletic performance. While acute inflammation is a necessary process for muscle repair and growth, chronic inflammation can be detrimental, hampering recovery and increasing the risk of injuries and illness. Various breathwork techniques, such as those focusing on prolonged exhales, have been shown to reduce markers of systemic inflammation. The reduced inflammation speeds up muscle recovery and mitigates the strain on other physiological systems like the cardiovascular and immune systems. This enables athletes to resume their training regimen with lesser downtime, contributing to a more consistent and productive athletic development cycle.

Furthermore, effective breathwork can reduce cortisol levels, the body's primary stress hormone. Elevated cortisol can lead to catabolism, where the body starts breaking down muscle tissue for energy, effectively undoing the gains from training. By managing cortisol through breathwork, athletes can protect against unwanted muscle breakdown, optimizing the anabolic processes necessary for muscle growth and improvement.

In essence, breathwork is an indispensable tool in the athlete's recovery arsenal. It allows for activating physiological states conducive to adequate rest, regeneration, and preparation for subsequent athletic challenges. Its benefits permeate through improved sleep, reduced inflammation, and better hormonal balance, making it an integral part of a well-rounded athletic regimen aimed at peak performance and sustainable health.

Breathwork offers a multi-faceted approach to both immediate performance enhancement and long-term well-being. As athletes aim to find that extra edge in their performance, the benefits of integrating breathwork into their daily training routines could be the game-changer they've been searching for. This practice warrants as much attention and discipline as any other element of an athlete's training, and those who master it will find themselves at a distinct advantage.

Yoga and Other Movement-based Practices

Yoga and other movement-based practices serve as more than just supplementary exercises for athletes; they act as multi-dimensional tools that positively impact various physical and mental well-being facets. These practices contribute to an athlete's mindfulness routine, a much-needed counterbalance to the often intense and highly focused nature of most athletic training.

Yoga's increasing ubiquity in the athletic world is far from coincidental. Its rich tapestry of poses, sequences, and breathing techniques can be personalized to meet each athlete's unique needs and objectives. This level of customization makes it a highly adaptable practice. The physical benefits, including increased flexibility, are manifold, and pivotal in preventing muscle strains and joint injuries. It also aids muscle recovery and can counteract the physical imbalances from sports that overuse particular muscle groups. Furthermore, yoga's focus on core strength and balance can enhance an athlete's power and stability, which are critical for almost every sport.

However, the benefits are more than merely physical. Yoga instills a sense of inner tranquility and mindfulness, fostering a deep mind-body connection. This psychophysiological synergy becomes a potent weapon in an athlete's arsenal, especially during high-pressure moments. Awareness of one's bodily sensations and mental states can lead to superior focus, greater resilience against stress, and enhanced decision-making during competitions.

Beyond yoga, other movement-based practices like Tai Chi and Qigong offer athletes substantial perks. Rooted in traditional

Chinese philosophy and medicine, these practices emphasize the flow of 'Qi' or life energy and aim to harmonize the body and mind. Tai Chi, often described as "meditation in motion," enhances balance, coordination, and proprioception—the sense of the relative position of one's body parts. Improved proprioception can result in superior technique and reduced risk of injury. With its focus on controlled breathing and fluid movement, Qigong can help athletes cultivate a focused mind and a relaxed, yet energized, body state.

Then there's dance, a movement-based practice that typically doesn't fall under traditional athletic training but offers substantial benefits nonetheless. Dance can improve agility, timing, and rhythm, which is particularly useful in sports requiring quick and coordinated movements. Moreover, dance cultivates artistic expression and emotional release, serving as an outlet for stress relief and psychological rejuvenation.

Integrating movement-based practices like yoga, Tai Chi, Qigong, and dance into an athlete's training regimen can offer a holistic approach to athletic development. By synergizing the physical enhancements with mental resilience and emotional stability, these practices create a well-rounded athlete capable of exceptional performance under various conditions. So, these practices are not merely add-ons but integral components that can significantly elevate athletic performance's physical and psychological aspects.

The Role of Mindfulness in Injury Prevention and Rehabilitation

The role of mindfulness in injury prevention and rehabilitation for athletes is multifaceted, touching on both the physical and psychological dimensions of well-being. It acts as both a proactive and reactive measure, aiding in not just averting injuries but also in the healing process should an injury occur.

From a prevention standpoint, mindfulness facilitates a heightened body awareness level often missing in traditional training programs. By continually tuning into their bodies, athletes can learn to discern even the subtlest signals of impending strain or fatigue, thus enabling them to make real-time modifications to their training routines or techniques. For example, a runner could use mindfulness techniques to become acutely aware of a slight discomfort in the knee, taking immediate steps to adjust form or even stop running altogether, thereby averting a more severe injury.

But it's not just about listening to the body; it's about heeding its messages. Mindfulness allows athletes to differentiate between "good" pain—the kind that signifies a productive workout—and "bad" pain that warns against potential damage. The internal dialogue cultivated through mindfulness equips athletes to make prudent decisions about pushing their limits or resting. This is especially crucial for those prone to overtraining and the resultant physical and psychological burnout.

Should an athlete sustain an injury, mindfulness doesn't lose its utility—it morphs into a different form of support. Anyone sidelined by an injury knows that the process isn't merely physically debilitating but emotionally draining. Here, mindfulness can act as a psychological salve. Techniques like meditation and breathwork come to the fore, aiding athletes in managing the emotional turbulence that often accompanies injury. By adopting a mindful approach, athletes can detach from negative emotions like frustration or impatience and view their situation from a stance of non-judgmental awareness. This mental clarity can aid in more rational decision-making about rehabilitation methods, engagement with healthcare professionals, and timelines for a safe return to activity.

Moreover, mindfulness can also be helpful during physical rehabilitation sessions. Whether an athlete is working through physical therapy exercises or easing back into training, maintaining a conscious, focused mind can enhance the body's healing capabilities. The athlete learns to listen and adapt, pace and persist, and this balanced approach can expedite recovery.

Mindfulness practices offer a holistic approach to injury prevention and rehabilitation. They augment the athlete's toolkit, providing physical, emotional, and psychological resources that can be vital in navigating the fraught landscape of athletic injuries. Therefore, the importance of such practices cannot be overstated as part of a well-rounded and effective athletic training program.

Building a Holistic Training Plan

The pursuit of athletic excellence requires a well-rounded and comprehensive approach to training. In this chapter, we will explore how to build a holistic training plan that incorporates traditional physical training methods and the use of magic mushrooms and mindfulness practices to support mental and emotional well-being. By adopting such an integrated approach, athletes can optimize their performance, minimize the risk of injury, and develop a deeper connection with their sport.

To create an effective training plan, addressing all aspects of an athlete's development, including physical conditioning, mental focus, and emotional resilience, is essential. Through traditional training techniques, the responsible use of magic mushrooms, and the incorporation of mindfulness practices, athletes can unlock their full potential and reach new heights in their athletic endeavors.

Integrating Magic Mushrooms into Your Existing Training Regimen

Balance and thoughtful experimentation are key when integrating magic mushrooms into an existing athletic training regimen. Magic mushrooms, whether consumed in micro or macro doses, serve distinct purposes and must be used judiciously to yield the most benefit while minimizing potential risks. This venture is as much a scientific endeavor as it is a holistic one, requiring strategic planning, timing, and attention to detail.

Starting with microdosing, the practice can be subtly powerful. Microdosing involves ingesting small, sub-perceptual amounts of magic mushrooms on a specific, carefully measured schedule, often every third or fourth day. This is less about inducing a radical alteration in consciousness and more about fine-tuning your existing cognitive and emotional frameworks. The doses are usually small enough to avoid a full-blown psychedelic experience, but substantial enough to produce a discernible shift in mental clarity, focus, and emotional well-being. Since athletes often require laser-sharp focus and a calm emotional state, microdosing can be a helpful tool. But it's not a one-size-fits-all; the optimal timing for microdosing can differ from one athlete to another. Some may find microdose on training days beneficial for that extra cognitive sharpness and emotional balance. In contrast, others might prefer to do it on rest days, facilitating mental recovery and providing a different type of preparation for the athletic challenges ahead.

Macrodosing, by contrast, is more intense and transformative, often reserved for addressing deeper psychological or emotional issues that could affect your performance. If you want to make significant mental shifts or overcome more substantial hurdles like performance anxiety or mental blocks, a macrodose could be appropriate. These sessions are not to be taken lightly and require careful planning. The 'set and setting,' meaning your mindset and the physical environment in which the experience occurs, are crucial for a safe and productive session. An athlete might choose to do this during the off-season or a break in training, as the recovery period afterward can be unpredictable.

Also, it's crucial to consider your sport or discipline's particular demands and objectives. For instance, endurance athletes may focus on how macrodosing could help them break through mental barriers related to physical fatigue. At the same time, a gymnast might explore how it could aid in achieving a greater sense of body awareness or spatial orientation. The questions you seek to answer or the aspects you aim to improve should guide your macrodosing sessions.

Thus, integrating magic mushrooms into your athletic routine requires more than just consuming the substance; it's a calculated endeavor requiring a blending of your physical training schedule, mental health needs, and performance goals. Whether microdosing to sharpen your day-to-day focus and emotional resilience or macrodosing to overcome more profound mental blocks, the key is to approach this integration with the same discipline, respect, and intentionality that you would apply to any other element of your athletic training.

Balancing Physical, Mental, and Emotional Well-being

A comprehensive approach to athletic training involves more than just improving physical performance; it also significantly emphasizes mental clarity and emotional resilience. Physical, mental, and emotional aspects are intrinsically linked, and optimizing one invariably impacts the others. So, when considering adding an unconventional component like magic mushrooms to your training regimen, viewing it as part of a broader, more balanced lifestyle that addresses various facets of well-being is imperative.

Physical health is, of course, a cornerstone. Without a well-conditioned body, even the best mental preparations can fall short. Therefore, focusing on a regimen that prioritizes rest and active recovery as much as it performs is essential. Implement stretching, foam rolling, or even gentle yoga sessions to expedite muscle recovery and alleviate physical stress. These practices can dovetail nicely with the effects of microdosing magic mushrooms, which some claim help to improve focus and speed up physical recovery.

However, an athletic career isn't just taxing on the body; it can be equally draining mentally. The constant pressure to perform and the ups and downs of competition can be mentally exhausting. That's where techniques like meditation and breathwork come in, serving as tools for mental hygiene. Stress management becomes a part of daily life, not an afterthought. Mindfulness practices, from journaling to visualization exercises, are crucial, helping you manage stress and maintain mental clarity that complements your physical conditioning.

Emotional well-being is the third pillar, often the most overlooked yet one of the most crucial. The emotional highs and lows accompanying competition require a solid support network for true resilience. Family, friends, and teammates who offer emotional nourishment can significantly impact long-term athletic success. Supplement this support by seeking professional help, like a sports psychologist or therapist, to dig deeper into emotional challenges that can hinder performance. With emotional resilience, the effects of microdosing magic mushrooms, like increased mood and emotional balance, can become even more beneficial.

Nutrition is the underpinning of all these facets of athletic performance. With proper fuel, both the body and the mind can continue. A balanced, nutrient-dense diet can offer the stamina needed for physical exertion and the cognitive sharpness required for split-second decisions. In the context of magic mushroom use, understanding the potential interactions between dietary choices and psychedelic experiences could be a critical area for further research and personal experimentation.

Finally, adopting a growth mindset can be a lynchpin for these elements. Embrace challenges as learning opportunities, recover from setbacks with increased vigor, and view obstacles not as hindrances but as chances for development. This mindset can be especially beneficial when integrating something as unconventional as magic mushrooms into your routine, as you'll be venturing into largely uncharted territory, rife with both challenges and opportunities.

Integrating magic mushrooms into a well-rounded training plan isn't just about the substance itself; it's about adopting a holistic approach that harmonizes physical prowess with mental clarity and emotional stability. By meticulously planning and integrating practices that foster each of these aspects, you prepare yourself for a level of athletic performance that is not just physically remarkable but also mentally and emotionally sustainable.

Developing a Personalized and Adaptable Plan

Creating a holistic training plan that seamlessly integrates the use of magic mushrooms necessitates a customized approach that accounts for your unique physiological and psychological makeup and your specific athletic goals. The first step in this personalized strategy involves thoroughly assessing your current fitness level. Evaluating your strengths, weaknesses, and areas in need of improvement will provide the foundational data you need to set achievable, realistic goals, both in the short-term and long-term. Once these goals are clearly outlined and broken down into smaller, trackable milestones, you can identify how the careful inclusion of magic mushrooms, either through microdosing or macrodosing, can amplify your training outcomes.

The following key consideration is thoughtfully including magic mushrooms into your plan. The goal is to complement and enhance your existing routine, not overpowering it. Thus, start conservatively and continually monitor your response, including any changes in physical performance, mental clarity, or emotional well-being. Adapt your approach based on these observations, ensuring you're always aligning with your broader training and well-being goals.

A well-rounded athletic regimen includes more than just one or two types of physical conditioning; it incorporates a blend of strength training, endurance work, skill development, and flexibility exercises. This diversity ensures that you are building muscle, enhancing your stamina, honing your athletic skills, and preventing injury through improved flexibility—factor in the necessary rest and active recovery periods to promote healing and muscle growth. The psychedelic experiences or focus enhancement facilitated by magic mushrooms should align with this balanced training methodology, not conflict with it.

A comprehensive strategy includes mental and emotional support resources alongside your physical training plan. These can range from mindfulness practices, like meditation or breathwork, to stress management techniques and even a reliable emotional support network consisting of friends, family, and professionals like sports psychologists. The emotional equilibrium and mental clarity that some report as benefits of magic mushroom use could synergize well with these other psychological and emotional support forms.

Monitoring and adaptability are your final yet perpetual steps. A static plan is a stagnant plan. Therefore, constantly review your strategies, track your progress, and make data-driven decisions to refine your approach. The effectiveness of magic mushrooms in aiding your athletic and mental performance is not a set-it-and-forget-it equation but a dynamic one, requiring ongoing adjustments in response to your evolving needs, findings, and external circumstances like competition schedules or life changes.

By crafting a plan that is both personalized and adaptable, you position yourself for the optimal athletic performance that is sustainable and holistic, taking into account not just your physical prowess but also your mental clarity and emotional resilience.

Tracking Progress and Adjusting as Needed

Consistent and precise tracking of your progress is not just a recommendation—optimizing a holistic training plan that incorporates magic mushrooms is necessary. One of the most effective ways to do this is to maintain a meticulous training journal. In this journal, note every detail of your workouts, from the exercises you do, the number of sets and repetitions, to the weight you lift. Additionally, it's crucial to log your experiences with magic mushrooms—dose sizes, timing, and any perceptible changes in your physical performance, mental focus, or emotional state.

Beyond journaling, setting regular self-check-ins is invaluable. Allocate time every week or month to step back and evaluate how closely you're inching toward your goals. Use these moments to honestly reflect on what's working, what's not, and what unforeseen challenges or obstacles have come your way. These insights become actionable data, enabling you to fine-tune your strategy effectively.

Moreover, while subjective feelings are crucial, complement them with objective measures for a fuller picture. Track personal records in your chosen athletic discipline, undergo regular body composition assessments, and consider other performance tests relevant to your sport. These metrics are concrete markers of your physical progress, providing quantifiable proof of whether your training and magic mushroom protocols serve their intended purpose.

Paying keen attention to your body's signals can't be overstated. The sensation during and after workouts, your general energy levels, mood, and even quality of sleep indicate whether you're on the path to overtraining or need to adjust your training or mushroom dosage.

Pay attention to the utility of external feedback too. Coaches, trainers, or even fellow athletes can provide a different but valuable perspective on your performance. They can point out areas you may be lacking, which could be particularly enlightening when you're too close to the process to view it objectively.

Lastly, flexibility in your approach is essential. No training plan should be set in stone, no matter how well-considered. Life changes, goals evolve, and new information may become available that could require changes to your training regimen or magic mushroom protocol. Embracing the need for adaptability rather than resisting it can be your greatest asset for continued growth and achievement in your athletic pursuits.

By employing these multi-faceted strategies for tracking and adapting, you're not just going through the motions; you're actively steering your athletic journey, enhancing your physical prowess and mental and emotional well-being.

Leveraging Digital Tools to Monitor and Optimize Your Holistic Athletic Training

In today's digitally connected world, optimizing athletic performance isn't solely about the sweat you pour into each training session; it's also about how you monitor, analyze, and adjust based on the data you collect. As you embark on a holistic athletic journey that integrates diverse strategies—from strength training and mindfulness practices to magic mushroom protocols—you must have the right tools at your fingertips to track your progress effectively.

Whether it's logging your physical workouts, assessing your mental and emotional state, or jotting down insights from your experiences with psychedelics, there's likely an app or digital platform tailored to your needs. This section will explore various digital tools designed to streamline the tracking process, making it easier for you to stay on course and achieve your athletic goals.

Tracking your progress becomes much more manageable and accurate when using digital tools designed specifically for that purpose. Here are some types of apps that can be particularly useful:

Fitness & Workout Tracking Apps

1. **MyFitnessPal**: Great for tracking nutrition, and exercise, and even has features to track macros for diet-conscious people.
2. **Strava**: Ideal for runners and cyclists, this app is excellent for tracking routes, pace, and elevation.
3. **JEFIT**: Good for gym-goers looking to log weightlifting exercises, sets, and reps.
4. **Fitbod**: Creates personalized workouts and tracks your lifting statistics.

Mindfulness and Mental Health Apps

1. **Headspace**: Offers guided mindfulness and meditation exercises.
2. **Calm**: Another meditation app that also includes sleep stories and breathing exercises.
3. **Smiling Mind**: Provides age-appropriate mindfulness exercises and has programs for athletic mindfulness.
4. **Insight Timer**: This has a vast library of free guided meditations and a customizable meditation timer.

General Health & Lifestyle

1. **Apple Health / Google Fit**: These native apps provide a broad range of tracking capabilities, from steps walked to hours slept.

2. **Whoop Strap**: Though not an app per se, this fitness tracker calculates strain, recovery, and sleep and syncs this data to an app on your phone.
3. **Garmin Connect**: If you use Garmin devices, this app helps consolidate all your health and fitness data in one place.

Sleep Tracking Apps

1. **Sleep Cycle**: Tracks the quality of your sleep and wakes you up during your lightest sleep phase.
2. **Oura Ring**: Again, not an app alone, but the Oura ring tracks various sleep metrics and provides them in an easy-to-understand format in its companion app.

Specialized Athletic Apps

1. **Coach's Eye**: You can record your physical movements (like a golf swing or a basketball shot) and analyze them to improve your form.
2. **Hudl**: Useful for team sports; lets you analyze video footage to improve team strategy.

Journaling Apps

1. **Day One**: A journaling app where you can log your personal reflections, training stats, or anything else.
2. **Journey**: Another versatile journaling app with cross-platform compatibility.

Each of these apps compiles valuable data that can inform your training decisions. When integrating magic mushrooms into your regimen, consider including a secure and private digital journaling option to track dosages and effects carefully. Continually assess how the tool fits into your strategy and adjust its use accordingly.

The Role of Sleep and Recovery in Performance

Athletic performance isn't solely dictated by the hours you spend lifting weights, running sprints, or honing your skills on the field. What happens after the training session is equally vital. In the quest for improvement, the role of sleep and recovery often takes a back seat, even though during these "off" hours, your body engages in the critical work of healing and building strength. During sleep, muscles repair, memories consolidate, and the mind refreshes, setting you up for the focus and mental agility needed in training and competition.

In this chapter, we are going more profound than just stating the importance of sleep. We'll explore the intricate relationships between sleep and the various physiological processes that are critical to athletic performance, from muscle recovery to cognitive function. Sleep isn't a monolithic entity; its quality, duration, and timing contribute to its effectiveness as a recovery tool. Therefore, understanding the nuances of sleep hygiene becomes pivotal for optimizing performance.

Furthermore, we'll delve into a unique angle—how magic mushrooms can influence sleep quality and accelerate recovery. While the intersection of psychedelics and sleep is still a burgeoning area of research, initial findings suggest a fascinating synergy that could be game-changing for athletes.

And we won't stop at just the "why"; this chapter will also equip you with actionable strategies to improve your sleep hygiene. We'll explore various techniques and interventions to help you fall asleep faster, sleep more deeply, and wake up refreshed. Finally, we will examine how sleep, training, and the thoughtful use of psychedelics can merge into a synergistic triad that might unlock new heights in your athletic pursuits.

By the end of this chapter, you'll have a comprehensive understanding of why prioritizing sleep is not just good practice but is an indispensable component of a holistic athletic performance strategy.

The Importance of Sleep for Athletes

Sleep is a vital component of an athlete's overall well-being and performance. During sleep, the body undergoes essential vital processes, such as muscle repair, immune system strengthening, and memory consolidation. Sleep is especially crucial for athletes due to the physical demands placed on their bodies during training and competition.

Several vital functions occur during sleep that directly impact an athlete's performance:

Muscle growth and repair: During deep sleep, the body releases growth hormones that facilitate muscle recovery and growth. This process is essential for athletes to build strength and resilience after intense training sessions.

Energy restoration: Sleep helps restore glycogen stores, the primary energy source for athletic performance. Adequate sleep ensures that athletes have the energy to perform at their best.

Cognitive function: Sleep is critical for maintaining optimal cognitive function, including memory, focus, and decision-making. These mental skills are essential for athletes who must react quickly and strategically in their respective sports.

Immune function: Sleep supports the immune system, which prevents illness and injury. Well-rested athletes are less likely to succumb to infections or experience setbacks due to injuries.

Sleep is a fundamental aspect of athletic performance, and neglecting it can hinder an athlete's ability to train, compete, and recover effectively.

How Magic Mushrooms May Influence Sleep Quality and Recovery

Magic mushrooms, containing the psychoactive compounds psilocybin and psilocin, may impact sleep quality and recovery for athletes. While research on this topic is still in its early stages, there are some potential ways in which magic mushrooms could influence sleep and recovery:

REM sleep enhancement: Some studies suggest that psilocybin may increase the duration of REM sleep, a crucial phase of sleep associated with dreaming, memory consolidation, and emotional regulation. Enhanced REM sleep could improve an athlete's mental and emotional well-being, contributing to better recovery and performance.

Sleep architecture: There is evidence that psilocybin can alter sleep architecture, potentially leading to sleep patterns and quality changes. However, more research is needed to determine the specific effects of psilocybin on sleep and whether these changes are beneficial or detrimental to athletic recovery.

Stress reduction: Magic mushrooms have been shown to reduce anxiety and stress, which can interfere with sleep quality. By alleviating stress, athletes may experience improved sleep, allowing them to recover more effectively from training and competition.

Mood regulation: Psilocybin has been found to positively affect mood and emotional well-being, which could indirectly impact sleep quality. Improved mood and emotional stability may contribute to better sleep, ultimately supporting recovery and performance.

It's important to note that the effects of magic mushrooms on sleep and recovery can vary among individuals, and more research is needed to understand these interactions fully. Athletes considering incorporating magic mushrooms into their recovery regimen should do so cautiously and under the guidance of a knowledgeable professional.

Sleep Hygiene and Strategies to Optimize Rest and Recovery

Sleep hygiene refers to the habits and practices that promote good sleep quality and daytime alertness. Optimizing sleep hygiene is crucial for enhancing recovery and overall performance for athletes. Here are some strategies to help athletes improve their sleep hygiene and optimize rest and recovery:

Establish a consistent sleep schedule: Going to bed and waking up simultaneously daily can help regulate the body's internal clock, promoting better sleep quality and daytime alertness.

Create a sleep-conducive environment: Make your sleep environment comfortable, quiet, and dark. Consider using blackout curtains, white noise machines, or earplugs to block out distractions and create a calming atmosphere.

Limit exposure to screens before bedtime: The blue light emitted by smartphones, tablets, and computers can interfere with the production of melatonin, a hormone that regulates sleep. Try to avoid screens for at least an hour before bed.

Develop a pre-sleep routine: Engage in relaxing activities, such as reading, meditation, or a warm bath, to signal your body that it's time to wind down and prepare for sleep.

Be mindful of caffeine and alcohol intake: Caffeine is a stimulant that can disrupt sleep if consumed too close to bedtime. In contrast, alcohol may help you fall asleep initially but can interfere with sleep quality later at night. Limit your consumption of these substances, especially in the hours leading up to bedtime.

Exercise regularly: Regular physical activity has been shown to improve sleep quality, but avoid intense exercise too close to bedtime, as it may interfere with your ability to fall asleep.

Manage stress: Incorporate stress-reduction techniques such as deep breathing, meditation, or yoga into your daily routine to help promote relaxation and improve sleep quality.

By adopting these sleep hygiene practices, athletes can enhance their rest and recovery, ultimately supporting better performance in training and competition.

The Connection Between Sleep, Training, and Psychedelic Use

Sleep, training, and psychedelic use interplay is complex and multifaceted. Sleep is vital to an athlete's recovery process, while training intensity and frequency can influence sleep quality. Psychedelics, particularly magic mushrooms, may also impact sleep patterns and overall recovery.

Sleep and training: Adequate sleep is essential for optimal athletic performance, as it supports muscle repair, immune function, and cognitive processes. Overtraining or intense training sessions close to bedtime can lead to difficulty falling asleep or disrupted sleep. Thus, it's essential to balance training load and schedule workouts in a way that promotes good sleep.

Psychedelic use and sleep: Psychedelics, including magic mushrooms, can influence sleep in various ways. Some users report enhanced sleep quality and vivid dreams, while others may experience difficulty falling asleep or disrupted sleep patterns. The impact of psychedelics on sleep may vary based on individual factors, dosage, and use timing. To minimize potential sleep disruptions, consider microdosing earlier or scheduling macrodosing sessions on days when adequate recovery time is available.

Optimizing recovery: To maximize the potential benefits of psychedelic use on athletic performance, it's crucial to prioritize sleep and recovery. Combining mindful psychedelic use with proper sleep hygiene, stress management, and a balanced training regimen can help athletes harness the potential benefits of magic mushrooms while minimizing any negative impacts on sleep and recovery.

By understanding the connection between sleep, training, and psychedelic use, athletes can make informed decisions about incorporating magic mushrooms into their performance-enhancement strategies while prioritizing rest and recovery for optimal results.

The Mental Aspects of Athletic Performance

As athletes strive for peak performance, it becomes increasingly evident that mental fortitude is crucial in determining success. The mental aspects of athletic performance encompass an array of factors, including mental toughness, resilience, a growth mindset, and the ability to overcome anxiety and self-doubt. In this part of the journey, we will explore the various dimensions of the mental game and how magic mushrooms can help athletes develop essential mental skills and enhance their mental performance.

Developing Mental Toughness and Resilience

Mental toughness and resilience are vital to an athlete's success, enabling individuals to persevere through challenges, setbacks, and failures. Developing mental toughness involves cultivating the ability to maintain focus, confidence, and motivation in adversity. Resilience, conversely, refers to the capacity to bounce back and recover from setbacks or disappointments quickly. Athletes can benefit from incorporating strategies to strengthen their mental toughness and resilience, such as setting clear goals, embracing challenges, practicing self-compassion, and learning from failure. Magic mushrooms, mainly through microdosing, may help athletes enhance their mental toughness and resilience by promoting a deeper connection to their inner resources and fostering a more adaptive response to stress and adversity.

Macrodosing can be a powerful tool for athletes seeking to develop mental toughness. When taken in larger doses, magic mushrooms can induce profound, immersive experiences that may challenge an individual's emotional and psychological boundaries. These experiences can push athletes out of their comfort zones and force them to confront their fears, insecurities, and perceived limitations.

During a macrodosing session, athletes may encounter difficult emotions or thoughts, face personal challenges, or confront past traumas. Navigating these experiences requires a certain degree of mental resilience and determination, which can help develop mental toughness. As athletes learn to face and overcome internal obstacles, they become better equipped to handle the challenges and setbacks they encounter in their athletic pursuits.

Moreover, the insights gained from a macrodosing experience can lead to shifts in perspective and a deeper understanding of the self, allowing athletes to recognize and address self-defeating thoughts and behaviors that may hinder their progress. By fostering self-awareness, introspection, and emotional resilience, macrodosing can help athletes cultivate the mental toughness needed to excel in their sport and achieve their full potential.

Using Magic Mushrooms to Cultivate a Growth Mindset

A growth mindset is the belief that one's abilities, intelligence, and talents can be developed through hard work, persistence, and dedication. This mindset is crucial for athletes, encouraging continuous learning, improvement, and adaptability. Magic mushrooms can play a role in cultivating a growth mindset by facilitating introspection, self-awareness, and the breaking down mental barriers that may be limiting progress.

Psilocybin, the active compound in magic mushrooms, has been shown to promote neuroplasticity and stimulate new neural connections, potentially fostering a more flexible and adaptive mindset. When controlled and intentional, magic mushrooms can help athletes challenge their limiting beliefs, reframe their perspectives on failure and setbacks, and embrace a more open and growth-oriented approach to their training and performance. By incorporating microdosing or macrodosing into their routines, athletes can leverage the psychological benefits of magic mushrooms to nurture a growth mindset and enhance their overall performance.

Overcoming Performance Anxiety and Self-doubt

Performance anxiety and self-doubt are common challenges faced by athletes at all levels. The pressure to perform well, high expectations, and the fear of failure, can lead to stress and hinder optimal performance. When used responsibly, magic mushrooms can help athletes address these issues and improve their mental game.

Through both microdosing and macrodosing, magic mushrooms can help athletes better understand their thought patterns and emotional responses. This self-awareness can enable them to recognize and address the root causes of their performance anxiety and self-doubt. By confronting and working through these underlying issues, athletes can develop a more positive mindset and a stronger belief in their abilities.

Also, magic mushrooms can encourage a sense of connection and oneness, which may help athletes feel more in tune with their bodies and environment. This heightened sense of presence and focus can make it easier for them to stay in the moment during competition, rather than being consumed by worry or self-doubt.

By incorporating mindfulness techniques, visualization exercises, and other mental training strategies alongside the responsible use of magic mushrooms, athletes can develop practical tools for overcoming performance anxiety and self-doubt, ultimately leading to enhanced performance and personal growth.

Techniques to Enhance Mental Performance

To complement the use of magic mushrooms in improving mental performance, athletes can employ various techniques that help them build mental strength, maintain focus, and cultivate a positive mindset. Some effective strategies include:

Affirmations: These are positive statements that athletes can repeat to themselves to reinforce self-belief and overcome negative thought patterns. By regularly reciting affirmations, athletes can instill confidence in their abilities and foster a more optimistic outlook.

Cognitive reframing: This technique changes how athletes perceive and interpret their thoughts and experiences. By consciously shifting their perspective, they can reframe negative thoughts or situations into more positive and empowering ones. This can help them maintain motivation and resilience in the face of challenges.

Visualization: Athletes can mentally rehearse their performance, imagining themselves executing their skills flawlessly and achieving their desired outcomes. This mental practice can help build confidence and improve focus during competition.

Mindfulness meditation: Regular meditation can help athletes cultivate self-awareness, emotional regulation, and mental clarity. By learning to stay present and focused on the task, they can minimize distractions and perform at their best.

Goal setting: Establishing clear, achievable goals can provide athletes with a sense of direction and motivation. By breaking down larger objectives into smaller, manageable steps, they can maintain a sense of progress and accomplishment throughout their training.

Progressive muscle relaxation: This technique helps athletes release muscle tension and promotes relaxation. By systematically tensing and relaxing different muscle groups, they can become more aware of bodily sensations and develop better control over their physiological responses, especially during high-stress situations.

Breathing exercises: Controlled breathing exercises can help athletes regulate their emotional state, reduce anxiety, and improve focus. By practicing slow, deep breaths, they can lower their heart rate and enter a more relaxed and focused state of mind.

Journaling: Keeping a journal can allow athletes to express their thoughts, feelings, and experiences. Reflecting on their progress, challenges, and achievements can help them gain valuable insights into their mental and emotional well-being, facilitating personal growth and self-awareness.

Gratitude practice: Regularly expressing gratitude can help athletes maintain a positive mindset and improve overall well-being. By focusing on what they are grateful for, they can develop a more optimistic outlook and enhance their mental resilience.

Developing a pre-performance routine: Creating a consistent pre-performance routine can help athletes prepare mentally and emotionally for competition. This routine may include visualization, affirmations, or breathing exercises, and can help them enter a focused and confident state of mind.

Athletes can further enhance their focus, motivation, and mental resilience by integrating these mental performance techniques with responsible magic mushroom use, improving performance and personal growth.

Using Microdosing and Macrodosing to Enhance Focus, Motivation, and Mental Resilience

Both microdosing and macrodosing magic mushrooms can play a significant role in improving an athlete's mental performance. When used responsibly and strategically, these approaches can complement traditional mental training techniques and offer unique benefits.

Microdosing can benefit athletes looking to enhance focus, motivation, and mental resilience. By taking small, sub-perceptual doses of magic mushrooms every few days, athletes may experience several positive effects on their mental performance:

Enhanced Focus: Microdosing has been reported to improve concentration and attention, allowing athletes to maintain focus during long training sessions or competitions. This increased focus can lead to more productive workouts and improved overall performance.

Increased Motivation: Athletes may find that microdosing helps boost their motivation and drive, making it easier to commit to rigorous training regimens and maintain a positive attitude. This can be particularly helpful during challenging periods, such as overcoming plateaus or dealing with setbacks.

Improved Mental Resilience: Microdosing can potentially support mental resilience by helping athletes cope with stress, anxiety, and self-doubt. With greater mental resilience, athletes can be better equipped to handle the pressures of competition and the emotional ups and downs of pursuing high-level athletic goals.

Strengthened Mind-Body Connection: Some athletes report that microdosing helps deepen their mind-body connection, enabling them to understand better and control their physical movements. This enhanced connection can improve technique, balance, and overall performance.

Heightened Body Awareness: Microdosing may increase an athlete's sensitivity to their body's movements, sensations, and limitations. This heightened body awareness can lead to improved technique, more efficient movement patterns, and a reduced risk of injury.

Enhanced Mental Stamina: Athletes who microdose may experience increased mental stamina, allowing them to maintain focus and concentration during long, demanding training sessions or competitions.

Faster Reaction Times: Some athletes report faster reaction times while microdosing, which can be particularly beneficial in sports that require quick decision-making and rapid adjustments, such as tennis, basketball, or soccer.

Improved Adaptability: Microdosing may help athletes more effectively adapt to changing circumstances and unexpected challenges during training or competition. This increased adaptability can lead to better overall performance and a greater ability to overcome setbacks.

Greater Mind-Muscle Connection: Microdosing may enhance the mind-muscle connection, enabling athletes to engage specific muscle groups more effectively and optimize their movements during training and competition.

Emotional Resilience: Microdosing can help athletes build emotional resilience, allowing them to more effectively cope with the stress and pressure associated with high-level sports performance.

Enhanced Creativity: Some athletes report increased creativity and problem-solving abilities while microdosing. This can be beneficial in sports that require strategic thinking, such as martial arts, chess, or team sports where players must adapt to constantly changing situations.

Incorporating microdosing into an athlete's routine may provide a range of benefits related to focus, motivation, and mental resilience, ultimately supporting their pursuit of peak performance.

Macrodosing, or taking larger doses of magic mushrooms, can also profoundly impact an athlete's focus, motivation, and mental resilience. While the experience can be more intense and potentially challenging, it may offer valuable insights and breakthroughs that support athletic performance:

Enhanced Self-Awareness: Macrodosing can facilitate a deep exploration of one's thoughts, emotions, and beliefs. This increased self-awareness can help athletes identify and address mental barriers or limiting beliefs hindering their performance.

Emotional Processing and Healing: A macrodosing session may bring to the surface unresolved emotions or past experiences that could affect an athlete's motivation and focus. By processing and healing these emotional wounds, athletes can free up more mental energy to devote to their training and performance.

Strengthened Mind-Body Connection: Macrodosing can also deepen the mind-body connection, allowing athletes to understand their physical movements and sensations better. This heightened awareness can improve technique, balance, and overall performance.

Personal Growth and Resilience: Navigating the challenges and insights that can arise during a macrodosing session can help athletes develop greater mental resilience and a growth mindset. This resilience can be carried over into their athletic pursuits, helping them persevere in adversity and focus on their goals.

Improved Flow State: Some athletes report that macrodosing can facilitate access to the "flow state" – a mental state in which an individual is fully immersed in an activity, leading to a heightened sense of focus, creativity, and optimal performance. Experiencing this state during a macrodosing session may provide insights into achieving and maintaining flow states in athletic contexts.

Enhanced Visualizations: Macrodosing can produce vivid and immersive visual experiences. Athletes can harness this heightened imaginative capacity to create mental images of their desired performance outcomes, reinforcing neural pathways associated with specific movements, techniques, and strategies.

Increased Motivation and Goal Setting: A profound macrodosing experience can bring clarity and renewed motivation to an athlete's training regimen. The reflective nature of the experience may help athletes reassess their goals, identify their intrinsic motivation, and develop a more significant commitment to achieving their objectives.

Overcoming Plateaus: Athletes often experience performance plateaus, where progress seems to stall despite consistent training. Macrodosing can help athletes identify and break through these plateaus by providing new perspectives, uncovering hidden mental barriers, and inspiring innovative approaches to training.

Boosting Self-Confidence: Macrodosing can foster a sense of unity and interconnectedness, making athletes feel more confident in their abilities and less fearful of failure. This increased self-confidence can translate to improved performance, as athletes are more likely to trust their instincts and push themselves to their full potential.

While macrodosing may not be suitable for all athletes or situations, it can offer a unique opportunity for personal growth and enhanced mental performance that ultimately supports athletic goals. It is essential to approach macrodosing responsibly and with proper preparation to maximize its potential benefits.

Both microdosing and macrodosing magic mushrooms can offer unique benefits to athletes seeking to improve their mental performance. By incorporating these practices into a comprehensive training program, athletes can develop a solid mental foundation that supports their physical abilities and contributes to overall success in their chosen sport.

Here are a few examples of how microdosing and macrodosing magic mushrooms could impact an athlete's mental performance:

A marathon runner struggling with motivation during training sessions might incorporate microdosing into their routine to increase focus and drive. By taking small, sub-perceptual doses of magic mushrooms every few days, the runner may find it easier to stay committed to their training goals and maintain a positive attitude throughout the process.

A tennis player experiencing performance anxiety during high-stakes matches could benefit from a macrodosing session during their off-season. By confronting and working through their fears in a safe, controlled environment, the athletes may gain valuable insights that help them remain calm and focused in pressure-filled situations.

A powerlifter with a mental block preventing them from reaching new personal records might explore microdosing to enhance their mental resilience. By taking small doses of magic mushrooms, the powerlifter could break through the mental barrier and approach their training with renewed confidence and determination.

A gymnast recovering from a significant injury might use a macrodosing session to address the emotional and psychological challenges associated with rehabilitation. The profound experiences during the session could help the gymnast accept their situation, let go of fear or self-doubt, and develop a more positive mindset as they work towards regaining their previous level of performance.

A basketball player struggling with team dynamics might incorporate microdosing into their routine to improve communication and collaboration. By taking small doses of magic mushrooms, the athlete may become more empathetic, allowing them to understand their teammates' perspectives better and foster a more cohesive team environment.

A swimmer experiencing a plateau in their performance could benefit from a macrodosing session to tap into their creative problem-solving abilities. By exploring new techniques or strategies during the session, the swimmer might discover innovative ways to refine their stroke or approach to training, ultimately leading to breakthroughs in performance.

A soccer player with self-doubt and negative self-talk might use microdosing to cultivate a growth mindset. By taking small, sub-perceptual doses of magic mushrooms, the athlete may find it easier to focus on the learning process and view setbacks as opportunities for growth rather than failures.

A track and field athlete coping with the mental challenges of returning to competition after a long break might benefit from a macrodosing session. The experience could help them confront lingering fears or anxieties and provide them with a newfound sense of purpose and motivation, enabling them to approach their training and competitions with renewed enthusiasm and determination.

A cyclist facing burnout from excessive training might use microdosing to regain balance and joy in their sport. By taking small doses of magic mushrooms, the cyclist could reconnect with the intrinsic pleasure of cycling and rediscover their passion for the sport, ultimately leading to a more sustainable and fulfilling athletic career.

These examples illustrate how microdosing and macrodosing magic mushrooms can support athletes in various sports by addressing specific mental challenges, enhancing focus, motivation, and resilience, and ultimately contributing to improved performance.

Addressing Injuries and Pain Management

As athletes push their bodies to the limit, injuries and pain are often an inevitable part of the journey. Learning to manage pain and address injuries effectively is essential for maintaining long-term health and achieving peak performance. In this chapter, we'll delve into the potential applications of magic mushrooms for pain perception and management and explore the benefits of microdosing and macrodosing for injury recovery. We'll also discuss complementary therapies that can be used in conjunction with psychedelics to support a holistic approach to injury treatment and prevention. Finally, we'll emphasize the importance of listening to your body and adjusting your training regimen to ensure optimal performance and well-being.

The Role of Magic Mushrooms in Pain Perception and Management

Magic mushrooms, which contain the psychoactive compound psilocybin, have been found to have a notable impact on pain perception and management. Research has shown that psilocybin may help modulate how the brain processes pain signals, making it a potentially valuable tool for athletes with chronic pain or injury-related discomfort.

One of the ways magic mushrooms are thought to influence pain perception is through their interaction with serotonin receptors, particularly the 5-HT2A receptor. Activation of this receptor has been linked to decreased pain perception and increased pain tolerance. Additionally, psilocybin has been shown to promote neuroplasticity and neurogenesis, possibly contributing to the brain's ability to manage pain signals better.

Another factor to consider is the potential psychological impact of magic mushrooms on an individual's perception of pain. The profound experiences and altered states of consciousness induced by psilocybin could lead to shifts in perspective, allowing athletes to approach pain with a more positive mindset or even view it as a challenge to overcome rather than a debilitating obstacle.

It's important to note that while magic mushrooms may help with pain management, they should not be used as a substitute for professional medical advice or treatment. Athletes should consult a healthcare professional before incorporating any new substance into their pain management plan.

The Potential Benefits of Microdosing and Macrodosing for Injury Recovery

When used responsibly, magic mushrooms may offer potential benefits for athletes seeking to enhance their injury recovery process. Both microdosing and macrodosing could have unique advantages for athletes facing different aspects of recovery.

Microdosing involves taking small, sub-perceptual doses of magic mushrooms every few days. This practice may help athletes maintain a positive mindset during recovery and potentially enhance their focus on rehabilitation exercises. By improving mental resilience and motivation, microdosing could contribute to a more effective and efficient recovery.

Macrodosing, on the other hand, involves taking larger doses of magic mushrooms, resulting in a more profound, psychedelic experience. These experiences may help athletes address the emotional and psychological challenges associated with injuries, such as fear, self-doubt, or frustration. By working through these emotions in a controlled environment, athletes can potentially develop a more positive attitude and mental resilience, which can be crucial in overcoming setbacks and regaining their previous level of performance.

It is essential to recognize that while magic mushrooms may offer some potential benefits, they should not be considered a standalone treatment for injuries. Athletes should always prioritize a well-rounded recovery plan that includes proper medical care, physical therapy, and rest. Furthermore, it's crucial to consult a healthcare professional before incorporating any new substance into a recovery plan.

Complementary Therapies for Injury Treatment and Prevention

In addition to the potential benefits of magic mushrooms for injury recovery, athletes can explore various complementary therapies to enhance their treatment and prevention efforts. These therapies can help address both the physical and psychological aspects of injury management:

Physical therapy: Working with a licensed physical therapist can help athletes develop a tailored rehabilitation program that targets specific areas of concern. Physical therapy can include strengthening exercises, mobility work, and techniques to improve movement patterns and prevent re-injury.

Massage therapy can help reduce muscle tension, improve circulation, and promote relaxation. Regular massage therapy sessions can accelerate recovery and improve overall well-being.

Acupuncture: This traditional Chinese medicine practice involves inserting thin needles into specific points on the body. Acupuncture may help reduce pain and inflammation and address the mental and emotional components of injury recovery.

Chiropractic care: Chiropractic adjustments can help realign the spine and joints, improving biomechanics and reducing pain. Chiropractic care can benefit athletes dealing with spinal alignment or joint function issues.

Mindfulness meditation: Incorporating mindfulness practices, such as meditation and breathwork, can help athletes manage stress, anxiety, and negative emotions associated with injury recovery. Developing a mindfulness practice may also improve mental resilience and focus during rehabilitation.

Nutritional support: Proper nutrition is essential for optimal recovery. Working with a sports nutritionist or dietitian can help athletes create a personalized nutrition plan to support healing, reduce inflammation, and maintain a healthy body weight during recovery.

These complementary therapies can be used with conventional medical treatments and rehabilitation programs, alongside the responsible use of magic mushrooms. It's essential to consult a healthcare professional before incorporating any new therapy into an injury recovery plan.

The Importance of Listening to Your Body and Adjusting Your Training Regimen

One of the most critical aspects of injury prevention and recovery is learning to listen to your body and adjust your training regimen as needed. Athletes must develop a keen sense of self-awareness and be willing to adapt their training in response to physical and mental cues. Here are some strategies for tuning into your body and making informed decisions about your training:

Keep a training journal: Documenting your workouts, including exercises, sets, reps, and any relevant notes about how you felt during and after the session, can provide valuable insights into patterns and trends that may indicate the need for adjustments.

Prioritize rest and recovery: Ensure that you're getting adequate sleep and allowing your body enough time to recover between workouts. If you notice a decline in performance or increased fatigue, consider increasing your rest days or implementing active recovery sessions.

Be mindful of pain and discomfort: While some degree of discomfort is expected during intense training, persistent pain or unusual sensations should not be ignored. If you experience pain, consult a healthcare professional to determine the cause and make necessary adjustments to your training.

Monitor your mental and emotional well-being: In addition to physical cues, pay attention to your mental and emotional state. If you're feeling burned out, stressed, or anxious, it may be time to reassess your training program and incorporate stress-reduction techniques, such as meditation or mindfulness practices.

Regularly reassess your goals: As you progress through your training, your goals may evolve. Continually reassess your objectives and make adjustments to your training program accordingly. This may involve modifying your exercise selection, intensity, volume, or frequency.

Consult with professionals: Seek the guidance of experienced coaches, trainers, and healthcare professionals to help you make informed decisions about your training regimen. Their expertise can be invaluable in identifying potential issues and developing effective injury prevention and recovery strategies.

By listening to your body and being willing to adjust your training regimen, you can minimize the risk of injury, optimize your athletic performance, and support overall well-being. Integrating magic mushrooms and other complementary therapies into your training plan can further enhance these efforts when done responsibly and under professional guidance.

Ethical and Legal Considerations

As athletes explore the potential benefits of using magic mushrooms to improve their performance, they must consider the ethical and legal implications surrounding their use. While psychedelics can offer valuable insights and physical enhancements, they may also raise questions about fairness in competition, adherence to rules and regulations, and the potential for adverse effects. This chapter will discuss the legal landscape of magic mushrooms and sports, the ethics of using psychedelics for performance enhancement, and the role of governing bodies and anti-doping agencies in regulating their use. We will also address potential drug interactions and contraindications that athletes should be aware of when considering incorporating magic mushrooms into their training regimen. Ultimately, athletes must balance their personal goals with sportsmanship, fair competition, and a commitment to the well-being of themselves and their fellow competitors.

Navigating the Legal Landscape of Magic Mushrooms and Sports

The legality of magic mushrooms varies significantly across different countries and states. In some regions, they are strictly prohibited; in others, their use may be decriminalized or even legal for medicinal purposes. Athletes considering incorporating magic mushrooms into their training regimen must be aware of the laws and regulations in their jurisdiction to avoid potential legal consequences.

Additionally, governing bodies in sports have specific rules regarding using performance-enhancing substances. Many athletic organizations and anti-doping agencies, such as the World Anti-Doping Agency (WADA), have banned psychedelic substances like psilocybin, the active compound in magic mushrooms, for athletes participating in competitions. Violating these rules may result in penalties, disqualification, or suspension from competition.

Athletes must stay informed about the changing legal landscape and the regulations their respective sports organizations impose. Compliance with the law and adherence to the rules of their sport should be a priority for any athlete considering using magic mushrooms for performance enhancement.

Testing for psilocybin, the active compound in magic mushrooms, is not as joint as testing for other drugs like cannabis or anabolic steroids. However, it is still possible for an athlete to be tested for psilocybin if there is suspicion of its use or if the athlete is participating in a competition governed by an organization that tests explicitly for psychedelic substances.

The body metabolizes Psilocybin into psilocin, the compound responsible for the psychedelic effects. Drug tests that screen for psilocybin and psilocin typically use urine samples, but blood and hair samples can also be used in some instances. The detection window for psilocybin in urine is relatively short, usually around 1-3 days after ingestion. However, the detection window can be longer in blood and hair samples, with hair samples potentially showing use for up to several months after ingestion.

Athletes need to be aware of the testing protocols and substances monitored by their respective sports organizations. If an athlete is found to have used a banned substance like psilocybin, they may face penalties, disqualification, or suspension from competition. To avoid these consequences, athletes should carefully consider the potential risks and legal implications of using magic mushrooms for performance enhancement.

The Ethics of Using Psychedelics for Performance Enhancement

Using psychedelics, such as magic mushrooms, for performance enhancement in sports raises several ethical questions. These questions revolve around fairness, safety, and the spirit of competition.

Fairness: One of the primary ethical concerns surrounding the use of performance-enhancing substances in sports is fairness. If an athlete uses magic mushrooms to gain a competitive edge, it can be argued that they have an unfair advantage over their competitors who are not using such substances. This undermines the level playing field central to the spirit of sports.

Safety: Another ethical consideration is the safety of using psychedelics for performance enhancement. While growing evidence suggests microdosing and macrodosing magic mushrooms can positively affect mental well-being and cognitive function, the long-term safety of using these substances in a sports context remains unclear. Encouraging athletes to use psychedelics to gain a competitive advantage may risk their health and well-being.

Spirit of competition: The use of psychedelics for performance enhancement can also be seen as going against the spirit of sports, which is based on the idea of athletes competing against each other using their natural abilities, hard work, and determination. Introducing substances that alter an athlete's mental state and potentially give them an advantage might be viewed as detracting from the purity of competition.

Informed consent and autonomy: Athletes should have the right to make informed decisions about their bodies, including the use of substances that may enhance their performance. However, the pressure to win and the desire for success can sometimes lead athletes to make choices that might not be in their best interests, especially when using substances with unclear safety profiles.

In conclusion, while there may be potential benefits associated with using magic mushrooms for athletic performance enhancement, it is essential to carefully weigh the ethical considerations surrounding their use in a competitive sports environment. This includes addressing issues of fairness, safety, and the spirit of competition, as well as respecting individual athletes' autonomy and informed consent.

Balancing Personal Goals with Sportsmanship and Fair Competition

Balancing personal goals with the principles of sportsmanship and fair competition is crucial when considering the use of magic mushrooms for athletic performance enhancement. The following points can help athletes and coaches navigate this delicate balance:

Abide by the rules: To maintain a level playing field, athletes should adhere to the rules set forth by their respective sports organizations, including regulations on using performance-enhancing substances. If magic mushrooms are banned or restricted by a governing body, using them to gain a competitive advantage would be unethical and against the spirit of sports.

Prioritize health and well-being: Athletes should always prioritize their long-term health and well-being over short-term gains. Before using magic mushrooms or any other performance-enhancing substance, it is essential to thoroughly research the potential risks and benefits and consult with medical professionals to make informed decisions.

Emphasize hard work and dedication: Athletic success is built on hard work, dedication, and commitment to one's chosen sport. Using magic mushrooms or other substances should be considered as a supplement for consistent training and effort.

Respect opponents: Good sportsmanship involves treating opponents with respect and acknowledging their skills and accomplishments. Athletes should focus on competing fairly, using their natural abilities, and not relying on substances to gain an unfair advantage.

Open dialogue and education: Coaches, trainers, and athletes should engage in open and honest discussions about using performance-enhancing substances, including the potential benefits and risks associated with magic mushrooms. Education and awareness are vital in helping athletes make informed decisions and promoting fair competition.

By balancing personal goals with sportsmanship and fair competition, athletes can strive for success while upholding the values that make sports an enriching and meaningful endeavor. This involves adhering to the rules, prioritizing health and well-being, emphasizing hard work, respecting opponents, and fostering open dialogue and education on performance-enhancing substances.

The Role of Governing Bodies and Anti-doping Agencies

Governing bodies and anti-doping agencies are critical in ensuring that sports remain fair, competitive, and safe for all athletes. Their responsibilities about magic mushrooms and other performance-enhancing substances include:

Establishing and enforcing rules: Governing bodies are responsible for setting the rules and regulations for their respective sports, including those related to using performance-enhancing substances. They are tasked with creating policies that promote fair competition and protect the health of athletes. This may involve banning or restricting the use of certain substances, including magic mushrooms, in competition.

Testing and monitoring: Anti-doping agencies, such as the World Anti-Doping Agency (WADA), are responsible for developing and implementing testing procedures to detect the use of banned or restricted substances among athletes. This includes testing for substances like psilocybin and psilocin, the active compounds in magic mushrooms. These organizations may conduct in-competition and out-of-competition testing to ensure athletes abide by the rules.

Education and awareness: Governing bodies and anti-doping agencies also play a vital role in educating athletes, coaches, and trainers about the potential risks and benefits of using various substances, including magic mushrooms. Raising awareness and promoting informed decision-making can help prevent the misuse of performance-enhancing substances and protect the integrity of sports.

Research and development: Anti-doping agencies are involved in ongoing research efforts to understand better the effects of different substances on athletic performance and health. This research can inform future policy decisions, including those related to using magic mushrooms in sports.

Sanctions and penalties: When athletes are found to have violated anti-doping rules, governing bodies and anti-doping agencies are responsible for imposing appropriate sanctions and penalties. These measures deter athletes from using banned substances and ensure that those who do face consequences for their actions.

By fulfilling these roles, governing bodies and anti-doping agencies contribute to maintaining a level playing field in sports and promoting the safety and well-being of all athletes. They ensure that rules are established and enforced, athletes are tested and monitored, education and awareness efforts are ongoing, research is conducted, and appropriate sanctions are applied when necessary.

Potential Drug Interactions and Contraindications

When using magic mushrooms, it is crucial to be aware of potential drug interactions and contraindications to ensure safety and minimize risks. Athletes considering using magic mushrooms for performance enhancement should be particularly cautious, as they may be taking other medications or supplements that could interact with psilocybin or psilocin.

Serotonergic medications: Psilocybin and psilocin primarily act on serotonin receptors in the brain. As a result, there is a potential for interaction with other medications that affect serotonin levels, such as selective serotonin reuptake inhibitors (SSRIs), serotonin-norepinephrine reuptake inhibitors (SNRIs), and monoamine oxidase inhibitors (MAOIs). These interactions may lead to a dangerous condition called serotonin syndrome, characterized by symptoms like confusion, agitation, rapid heart rate, and high blood pressure.

Blood pressure medications: Magic mushrooms can cause transient increases in blood pressure, and combining them with medications may lead to unpredictable effects on blood pressure levels.

Stimulants: Combining magic mushrooms with stimulants like caffeine, amphetamines, or other performance-enhancing drugs may increase the risk of adverse side effects, such as elevated heart rate, anxiety, and overstimulation.

Sedatives and anti-anxiety medications: Magic mushrooms may interact with sedatives and anti-anxiety medications, leading to an increased risk of drowsiness or impaired coordination. This could be particularly dangerous for athletes who require high alertness and motor control during competition.

Other psychoactive substances: Combining magic mushrooms with other psychoactive substances, such as alcohol or recreational drugs, can lead to unpredictable effects and an increased risk of adverse reactions.

Athletes need to consult with a healthcare professional before using magic mushrooms, especially if they are taking any medications or supplements. A thorough understanding of potential drug interactions and contraindications can help minimize risks and ensure a safe, responsible approach to performance enhancement.

Conclusion

As we reach the end of our exploration into the potential of magic mushrooms for athletic performance, it is clear that these powerful substances hold immense promise for athletes seeking to push the boundaries of their physical and mental capabilities. The fusion of ancient wisdom and modern science has opened up new avenues for understanding and harnessing the power of psychedelics in sports and training.

The journey has only just begun, and the importance of continued research and exploration cannot be overstated. As we uncover more about the complex interactions between magic mushrooms and athletic performance, we will be better equipped to harness their potential benefits while minimizing risks and ensuring safety.

Responsible and informed use is crucial for the future of psychedelics in sports. Athletes, coaches, and researchers must work together to develop best practices, guidelines, and educational resources to promote these substances' safe and ethical use in the pursuit of athletic excellence.

The future of psychedelics in sports and training is full of possibilities, from enhancing mental resilience and focus to aiding recovery and injury management. As we continue to push the limits of human performance, we must remain open-minded, curious, and responsible in exploring these powerful tools. The potential for magic mushrooms to transform the world of athletics is only beginning to reveal itself, and the journey ahead promises to be exciting.

As the use of magic mushrooms in sports continues to evolve and gain more acceptance, it is essential to consider the next steps in this journey. Here are some areas that we should focus on in the future:

Education and awareness: To ensure the responsible and informed use of magic mushrooms in sports, it is essential to spread accurate information and provide education on the potential benefits and risks associated with their use.

Collaboration between researchers and athletes: To advance our understanding of how magic mushrooms can enhance athletic performance, researchers and athletes should collaborate on studies and share their experiences and insights.

Development of best practices and guidelines: As more athletes begin incorporating magic mushrooms into their training regimens, it will be essential to establish best practices and guidelines that ensure safety, efficacy, and ethical use.

Advocacy for policy changes: In many countries, magic mushrooms are still classified as illegal. Advocating for changes in policy and regulation could help make these substances more accessible for research and responsible use in sports.

Exploration of other psychedelics: Magic mushrooms are just one of many psychedelic substances with potential applications in sports. Future research should explore the effects of other psychedelics, such as LSD, ayahuasca, or DMT, on athletic performance.

Development of specialized products and services: As the use of magic mushrooms in sports becomes more mainstream, there will be opportunities for companies to develop specialized products and services tailored to the unique needs of athletes using these substances.

By focusing on these areas, we can continue to expand our understanding of the potential applications of magic mushrooms in sports and help athletes safely and effectively harness their benefits.

In conclusion, using magic mushrooms and other psychedelics in sports and athletic training can potentially revolutionize how we approach performance enhancement. The growing body of research on the topic suggests that these substances may offer unique physical, mental, and emotional benefits. However, it is crucial to approach their use with caution and responsibility, carefully considering the potential risks and ethical implications involved.

As we learn more about the synergistic effects of magic mushrooms with other performance-enhancing substances, athletes, and coaches will be better equipped to develop personalized and holistic training plans that maximize their potential. At the same time, promoting fairness and integrity in sports competitions is essential, ensuring that all athletes have equal access to safe and effective performance-enhancing methods.

By fostering open dialogue, supporting continued research, and advocating for responsible and informed use, we can help shape the future of psychedelics in sports and training positively and meaningfully. With a deepened understanding of these powerful substances, we can unlock new levels of human performance and push the boundaries of what is possible in sports.

Appendix: Resources and Further Exploration

Books and Articles

1. "Stealing Fire: How Silicon Valley, the Navy SEALs, and Maverick Scientists Are Revolutionizing the Way We Live and Work" by Steven Kotler and Jamie Wheal
2. "The Psychedelic Explorer's Guide: Safe, Therapeutic, and Sacred Journeys" by James Fadiman
3. "How to Change Your Mind: What the New Science of Psychedelics Teaches Us About Consciousness, Dying, Addiction, Depression, and Transcendence" by Michael Pollan
4. "The Third Wave: An Entrepreneur's Vision of the Future" by Paul Austin
5. "The Science of Microdosing Psychedelics" by Torsten Passie

B. Websites and Online Forums

1. The Third Wave (https://thethirdwave.co/)
2. Erowid (https://www.erowid.org/)
3. Shroomery (https://www.shroomery.org/)
4. Psychedelic Science (https://www.psychedelicscience.org/)
5. The DMT Nexus (https://www.dmt-nexus.me/)

C. Workshops and Retreats

1. Synthesis Retreat (https://www.synthesisretreat.com/)
2. MycoMeditations (https://www.mycomeditations.com/)
3. Soltara Healing Center (https://soltara.co/)
4. The Beckley Foundation (https://www.beckleyfoundation.org/)

5. The Psychedelic Society
   (https://psychedelicsociety.org.uk/)

D. Professional Organizations and Advocacy Groups

1. Multidisciplinary Association for Psychedelic Studies
   (MAPS) (https://maps.org/)
2. The Beckley Foundation
   (https://www.beckleyfoundation.org/)
3. The Psychedelic Society
   (https://psychedelicsociety.org.uk/)
4. The Heffter Research Institute
   (https://www.heffter.org/)
5. The Usona Institute (https://www.usonainstitute.org/)

These resources can provide valuable information, support, and guidance for those interested in exploring the potential of magic mushrooms and other psychedelics for athletic performance. However, it is essential to approach these resources with a critical mindset and remember that personal experiences and responses to psychedelics can vary significantly. Always prioritize safety, responsibility, and informed decision-making in your exploration of psychedelics and athletic performance.

References

1. Bogenschutz, M. P., & Johnson, M. W. (2016). Classic hallucinogens in the treatment of addictions. Progress in Neuro-Psychopharmacology and Biological Psychiatry, 64, 250-258. https://doi.org/10.1016/j.pnpbp.2015.03.002

2. Carhart-Harris, R. L., Bolstridge, M., Rucker, J., Day, C. M. J., Erritzoe, D., Kaelen, M., ... & Nutt, D. J. (2016). Psilocybin with psychological support for treatment-resistant depression: an open-label feasibility study. The Lancet Psychiatry, 3(7), 619-627. https://doi.org/10.1016/S2215-0366(16)30065-7

3. dos Santos, R. G., Bouso, J. C., & Hallak, J. E. (2017). Ayahuasca, dimethyltryptamine, and psychosis: a systematic review of human studies. Therapeutic Advances in Psychopharmacology, 7(4), 141-157. https://doi.org/10.1177/2045125316689037

4. Fadiman, J. (2011). The psychedelic explorer's guide: Safe, therapeutic, and sacred journeys. Simon and Schuster.

5. Griffiths, R. R., Johnson, M. W., Carducci, M. A., Umbricht, A., Richards, W. A., Richards, B. D., ... & Klinedinst, M. A. (2016). Psilocybin produces substantial and sustained decreases in depression and anxiety in patients with life-threatening cancer: A randomized double-blind trial. Journal of Psychopharmacology, 30(12), 1181-1197. https://doi.org/10.1177/0269881116675513

6. Grob, C. S., Danforth, A. L., Chopra, G. S., Hagerty, M., McKay, C. R., Halberstadt, A. L., & Greer, G. R. (2011). Pilot study of psilocybin treatment for anxiety in patients with advanced-stage cancer. Archives of General Psychiatry, 68(1), 71-78. https://doi.org/10.1001/archgenpsychiatry.2010.116

7. Hutten, N. R. P. W., Mason, N. L., Dolder, P. C., & Kuypers, K. P. C. (2019). Self-rated effectiveness of microdosing with psychedelics for mental and physical health problems among microdosers. Frontiers in Psychiatry, 10, 672. https://doi.org/10.3389/fpsyt.2019.00672

8. Johnson, M. W., Griffiths, R. R., Hendricks, P. S., & Henningfield, J. E. (2018). The abuse potential of medical psilocybin according to the 8 factors of the Controlled Substances Act. Neuropharmacology, 142, 143-166. https://doi.org/10.1016/j.neuropharm.2018.05.012

9. Kotler, S., & Wheal, J. (2017). Stealing fire: How Silicon Valley, the Navy SEALs, and maverick scientists are revolutionizing the way we live and work. HarperCollins.

10. MacLean, K. A., Johnson, M. W., & Griffiths, R. R. (2011). Mystical experiences occasioned by the hallucinogen psilocybin lead to increases in the personality domain of openness. Journal of Psychopharmacology, 25(11), 1453-1461. https://doi.org/10.1177/0269881111420188

11. Multidisciplinary Association for Psychedelic Studies (MAPS). (n.d.). https://maps.org/

12. Nichols, D. E. (2016). Psychedelics. Pharmacological Reviews, 68(2), 264-355. https://doi.org/10.1124/pr.115.011478

13. Pollan, M. (2018). How to change your mind: What the new science of psychedelics teaches us about consciousness, dying, addiction, depression, and transcendence. Penguin Press.

14. Prochazkova, L., Lippelt, D. P., Colzato, L. S., Kuchar, M., Sjoerds, Z., & Hommel, B. (2018). Exploring the effect of microdosing psychedelics on creativity in an open-label natural setting. Psychopharmacology, 235(12), 3401-3413. https://doi.org/10.1007/s00213-018-5049-7

15. Ross, S., Bossis, A., Guss, J., Agin-Liebes, G., Malone, T., Cohen, B., ... & Schmidt, B. L. (2016). Rapid and sustained symptom reduction following psilocybin

treatment for anxiety and depression in patients with life-threatening cancer: a randomized controlled trial. Journal of Psychopharmacology, 30(12), 1165-1180. https://doi.org/10.1177/0269881116675512

16. Stamets, P. (2005). Mycelium running: How mushrooms can help save the world. Ten Speed Press.

17. Studerus, E., Kometer, M., Hasler, F., & Vollenweider, F. X. (2011). Acute, subacute and long-term subjective effects of psilocybin in healthy humans: a pooled analysis of experimental studies. Journal of Psychopharmacology, 25(11), 1434-1452. https://doi.org/10.1177/0269881110382466

18. Swanson, L. R. (2018). Unifying theories of psychedelic drug effects. Frontiers in Pharmacology, 9, 172. https://doi.org/10.3389/fphar.2018.00172

19. The Beckley Foundation. (n.d.). https://www.beckleyfoundation.org/

20. The Heffter Research Institute. (n.d.). https://www.heffter.org/

21. The Third Wave. (n.d.). https://thethirdwave.co/

22. Usona Institute. (n.d.). https://www.usonainstitute.org/

23. Yaden, D. B., & Griffiths, R. R. (2018). The subjective effects of psychedelics are necessary for their enduring therapeutic effects. ACS Pharmacology & Translational

THANKS FOR READING

Thank you for diving into "The Athlete's Trip"! We hope it has broadened your perspective on the innovative use of magic mushrooms for athletic performance and personal excellence.

To further your exploration and connect with others on this unique journey, we invite you to visit trueeira.com/micro and claim your exclusive free gift, designed to enhance your athletic and personal development journey.

As you continue to push the boundaries of your capabilities, we'd be grateful if you could share your experiences by leaving a review. Your insights not only guide others in their pursuit of excellence but also contribute to the evolving narrative of performance enhancement and holistic well-being.

We value your involvement with the True Eira community and are excited to support you on your ongoing journey towards achieving peak performance and discovering your full potential.

Visit

trueeira.com/test

Find Your Microdose Personality

TRUE
EIRA

OUR MISSION

At True Eira, we are passionately committed to empowering athletes and individuals seeking to push the boundaries of their capabilities. Our focus is to provide a unique blend of traditional athletic training methodologies with groundbreaking practices, including the responsible use of magic mushrooms for enhancing performance and overall well-being.

Our mission is centered on more than just physical prowess; it encompasses a holistic approach to peak performance. We are dedicated to nurturing mental resilience and emotional balance, integral components of personal excellence. By melding the deep-rooted wisdom of established athletic disciplines with the transformative potential of modern scientific research, we offer comprehensive resources tailored to the needs of forward-thinking individuals.

True Eira aspires to create an environment that not only fosters greater athletic achievements but also supports each individual's journey of self-discovery and personal growth. Our goal is to bridge the gap between time-honored methods and cutting-edge techniques, contributing to the evolution of the athletic community. We strive to be a catalyst in this realm, inspiring and supporting a diverse group of individuals united in their quest to explore and expand the limits of human potential.

TRUE EIRA ORIGINS

In the heart of True Eira lies the transformative journey of its founder, Travis Eric. Inspired by his life-changing encounters with entheogens, Travis envisioned a path for a broader community seeking to unlock their full potential. He saw these ancient substances as tools for personal enlightenment and keys to unlocking a deeper understanding of human capability.

Travis created True Eira to build a platform where the ancient wisdom of entheogens could be harmonized with the pursuits of modern athleticism and personal development. He envisioned True Eira as a conduit for collective growth, a place where individual journeys towards self-discovery and peak performance could be nurtured and celebrated.

Travis assembled a team of researchers and experts to bring this vision to life. Together, they delved into entheogens' scientific and holistic aspects, exploring their myriad benefits and applications. This collaboration was grounded in a shared belief in the power of community in the pursuit of knowledge and self-improvement.

True Eira is a movement towards exploring the limits of human potential. It stands as an evolving entity, shaped by the contributions and discoveries of its community. Here, the journey of self-discovery is amplified by collective wisdom, where each member plays a role in shaping a future where the full spectrum of human potential is realized.

As True Eira moves forward, it carries the spirit of collaboration and exploration. It represents a space where minds meet and horizons expand, all united by the quest to discover what truly lies within and beyond the bounds of human capability.

THE ESSENCE OF TRUE EIRA

The name "True Eira" holds deep significance, inspired by Eir (or Eira), the Norse goddess of healing. In Norse mythology, Eira is known for her wisdom and expertise in healing and medicine, often associated with physical and spiritual well-being. By invoking the essence of Eira, we aim to embody her healing spirit and create a space that facilitates growth, self-discovery, and personal transformation.

The term "True" in our name signifies our commitment to authenticity and integrity in exploring the vast potential of human growth and self-discovery. We strive to provide reliable, research-based information and resources while honoring the ancient traditions that have long recognized the healing powers of various practices, including using entheogens.

Combining Eira's healing essence with our dedication to authenticity, the name "True Eira" represents our mission to empower individuals on their journey towards self-discovery, healing, and personal growth through a holistic approach, encompassing ancient and modern wisdom practices.

TRUE
E I RA

Customers Who Bought This Book Also Bought

Microdosing Magic: Unveiling the Transformative Power of Psychedelic Mushrooms

Healing Trauma with Magic Mushrooms: A Comprehensive Guide to Microdosing and Macrodosing Psilocybin for PTSD

Visit

trueeira.com/test

Find Your Microdose Personality

TRUE
EIRA